The handbook of residential care

D1376049

Based on the author's long and varied experience, *The Handbook of Residential Care* brings together all areas of residential work, and all levels of involvement in it. Throughout the book there is a unique combination of real examples, analysis, guidance and reflective discussion, so that reading the book parallels the process of doing the work – whether you are a basic grade practitioner, a student, a team leader, a manager, an inspector, a planner, or a management committee member or local politician.

At whatever level of involvement with residential care this book facilitates understanding both about face-to-face work with residents *and* about the workings and politics of organisations. Designed as a practical guide, it includes many examples of everyday experiences, which can be used as case studies in training. With its emphasis on direct personal work, the *Handbook* will promote effectiveness among residential workers – through self-management, building relationships, creating helpful organisation, and resisting bureaucratic and impersonal organisation.

Invaluable to all practitioners, team leaders and managers in residential care, the *Handbook* provides a wealth of new ideas and many challenges to established policy and practice.

John Burton has many years' experience as a residential worker – doing the work, managing it, thinking and writing about it, and helping to improve practice as a consultant and trainer.

084197

The handbook of residential care

John Burton

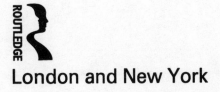

London and New York

First published 1993
by Routledge
11 New Fetter Lane, London EC4P 4EE

Simultaneously published in the USA and Canada
by Routledge
29 West 35th Street, New York, NY 10001

© 1993 John Burton

Typeset in Times by Michael Mepham, Frome, Somerset
Printed and bound in Great Britain by
Mackays of Chatham PLC, Chatham, Kent

British Library Cataloguing in Publication Data
A catalogue record for this book is available from the British
Library.

Library of Congress Cataloging in Publication Data
Burton, John, 1947–
    The handbook of residential care/John Burton.
    p.   cm.
    1. Institutional care–Great Britain.   I. Title.
    HV63.G7B87   1993
    362'.0425–dc20   93–14836
                                                                     CIP

ISBN 0–415–08635–3 (hbk)
       0–415–08636–1 (pbk)

To E. B. with love

Contents

List of figures   ix
List of examples   x
List of checklists   xii
Preface   xiii
Acknowledgements   xviii

Introduction   **1**

1   Scenes from residential work   **4**
Struggling to care   4
Complicated, exhausting work   7
Arguing with Bertram   13
Preparing tea   16
Local politics   19

2   Understanding and managing: making a start   **23**
Starting work   23
Applying self-management   28
The working use of principle   32
Organising yourself   35

3   Giving and receiving   **41**
Fantasy/Phantasy, the unconscious, transference and
    counter-transference   41
Building and using relationships   42
Building relationships with children   48
Bedtime   52
Physical assistance: bathing   56
Sexuality   58
Control   64
The rewards of the job: giving and receiving   69

4   Leading and influencing: creating and using vision   72
Vision   72
Management and leadership: a reassessment   73
Sharing responsibility   78
Becoming a senior worker   80

5   Creating helpful organisation   90
It's not so much the building as the way you use it   90
Inclusion/exclusion   97
Food and catering   100
Staff organisation   102
Supervision   105
Training and development   109
Rotas   111
Routines, rules and habits   114

6   Resisting hindering organisation   124
Organisation(s)   124
Organisations as systems   125
The role of the manager   136
The policy roundabout   138

7   Outside assistance   144
What is an outsider?   145
The roles of outsiders   148

8   A good place to live?   157
*Boundaries are important but broken rules aren't the end
  of the world: Joe's story*   158
Packed off and forgotten: Theresa's story   160
*If I'm good they're going to keep me; if I'm bad they're
  going to move me: Sandra's story*   164
*I chose to come here; I manage well:
  Mrs Dunsford's story*   167

9   Liberating institutions: a future for residential care   169
Past, present and future   169
Exploiting the bandwagon of superficial change   180

Appendix 1 The learning basket   186
Appendix 2 Change   188
Appendix 3 Models, images and cultures of
  organisations, establishments, units, homes and teams   190
Bibliography   193
Index   197

Figures

4.1 Three management styles 76

4.2 Expectations of Supermanager 80

6.1 An organisation as a socio-technical system 126

6.2 A residential home as a socio-technical system 128

6.3 A hindering organisation 130

6.4 A residential establishment as an outpost of a
bureaucratic organisation 133

6.5 A large organisation as three defensive systems 134

A1 The learning basket 186

A2 An image and some ideas about different levels of
change and resistance to change 188

Examples

2 Understanding and managing

2.1 Being unreliable   29

2.2 A residential management group   35

2.3 Using a diary   37

3 Giving and receiving

3.1 Dusty Miller: an emergency admission   42

3.2 Making bedtime a therapeutic time   53

3.3 A relationship between a worker and a resident   60

3.4 A young man working with teenage girls   63

3.5 Using physical force to hold a child   66

3.6 Women with authority   67

4 Leading and influencing

4.1 A care worker's vision   72

4.2 A resident's vision   73

4.3 The domestic worker and the director   74

4.4 Buying food in a bureaucracy   78

4.5 Sharing responsibility for food   78

4.6 The experience of becoming a manager appointed
     from outside   82

4.7 Promotion from within   85

5 Creating helpful organisation

    5.1 Involving everyone in changing the home   91

    5.2 A significant sideboard   95

    5.3 Every picture tells a story   96

    5.4 A purposeful network of meetings   103

    5.5 A training and development culture   109

    5.6 Getting to grips with a delinquent subculture   118

    5.7 Religion and culture: bad practice   123

6 Resisting hindering organisation

    6.1 The kitchen cupboard list   131

    6.2 Organisational response to scandal   138

7 Outside assistance

    7.1 Visitors not admitted   147

    7.2 Picking up clues and taking action   149

9 Liberating institutions

    9.1 Charity and politics in a children's home   171

    9.2 Acre Lane Community Care Centre: a vision of the
         future   175

    9.3 Taking the initiative and making practical changes   182

Checklists

2 Understanding and managing
Understanding yourself in this job   27
Understanding the job   28
Self-analysis/awareness   30
Tips for reliability   32
Managing with principle   33
Managing your own work   39

3 Giving and receiving
Building and using relationships   51
Bedtime checklist   55
Giving intimate care   57
The rewards of residential work   70

4 Leading and influencing
Becoming a manager   86

5 Creating helpful organisation
Checklist for staff meetings   105
Some useful tips for supervisors   107
Constructing a rota   112

6 Resisting hindering organisation
Checklist for resisting hindering organisation   142

Preface

In September 1965 I was sent to live in a probation hostel in Paddington. I was one of the early Community Service Volunteers (CSV), just starting to get to grips with the most important part of my education. By day I learned under the guise of being an assistant to an inspiring teacher who taught the Social Education classes at North Paddington Upper School. Most of the rest of my time was spent in the hostel – almost literally a 'den of thieves', which was how Mrs P, the cook, described it to me the day I arrived.

I remember my arrival well. I had been in London only once before, briefly. Wearing a grey suit and carrying a large new suitcase, both of which my mother had given me before leaving home, I stepped out of the taxi I had taken from the station. I had expected that the accommodation which Alec Dickson, then the director of CSV, had arranged for me would provide me with my own room and access to a shared bathroom and kitchen. My expectations were soon shaken when I was greeted at the door by Pete, a stout, unshaven man of indeterminate age, who ushered me into the dark interior. I was quickly introduced to Mrs P whose first question was to ask what it was that I had done to land up there. I simply didn't understand her but after an uncomfortable gap during which Mrs P stared at Pete, she suddenly exclaimed, 'Of course, you're John!' and told me to be careful. I was no wiser but more anxious and confused as I hauled my suitcase up the dark stairs, followed by Pete asking me if I had any valuables which I would like to leave with him. I didn't even know who Pete was and I said that I was sure that my things would be safe in my locked suitcase. We passed a large room on the first floor with the open door revealing a sofa with two of its legs missing and a TV flickering and blaring in the corner. There were people in the room and their loud argument outdid the television in volume. 'The lounge,' said Pete. 'I'll introduce you to the lads later.'

We passed a room on a half-landing; 'The shower,' motioned Pete. We continued to climb, my suitcase lurching against the unsteady bannisters and a vaguely unpleasant smell becoming a strong stink of cats. The loose and frayed stair carpet had given way to bare, rough boards.

'Here you are,' said Pete, pushing open a door. 'Right at the top. You can have either of these two beds; they're both free.' There were four iron bedsteads in the room. The two offered to me both had striped unsprung mattresses, stained in the middle by bed-wetting former occupants. A meagre pillow was at one end of each and a pile of coarse brown blankets at the other. There was barely space for the four beds, four bedside cabinets, a chest of drawers and a built-in wardrobe. One small window looked out on to a parapet wall and over the roofs of the opposite houses.

I lived at the hostel for about four months. It was a risky but very proper, even inspired, decision to send me there. Had I been offered a choice, I would have chosen somewhere more comfortable and less personally challenging. There is much that is vividly memorable about that time for me, not least my 'admission' to a residential institution and the lives of my fellow residents. The deep deprivation was a shock to me; every sense and feeling was starved or abused. I can remember the disorientation I experienced on visiting my own home during the first half-term and picking up a clean glass, stroking my hand across polished wood, being on my own in a room in a quiet house, and feeling that this and the hostel were two separate worlds. As Pete had predicted and attempted to pre-empt, my 'valuables', principally my camera, were stolen by someone who had become a friend and who returned to prison after the concentrated spree of housebreaking which started with stealing from me.

My work at the school was equally disturbing – and educational – for me. I had two exceptional teachers. One appeared to like and believe in every deprived and difficult fourteen- or fifteen-year-old who was allocated to her classes on grounds of low attainment, a low IQ score or bad behaviour, and gave each of them trust and respect for themselves. The other, one of the very few Black teachers on a large staff in a multiracial school, simply took me under his wing. My adolescent White liberalism was adamantly integrationist and colour-blind, and I could see little of the racism that was all around me and deeply within myself. With Frank's great help and tolerance, and, I suspect, his almost anthropological interest, I began to learn.

The children I worked with, fourteen- and fifteen-year-olds, some of whom were considerably more mature and wordly wise than me, also contributed to my social education as we discovered London together, made a film, dug the hospital garden and engaged in the many unusual educational activities which Raechel, our inspiring and optimistic teacher and mentor, thought might be useful and interesting fun. In return, I taught two children to read and tried to teach several more.

In 1966 I got a job with Task Force (now Pensioners' Link) and then went to work at another school, Tulse Hill in Brixton. In retrospect, both were significant moves and besides continuing my late education probably contributed to my later involvement in work with older people and to my becoming a long-time resident of Brixton.

Brent Children's Reception Centre in 1968 was my first proper residential job. (It was later to move to a new building and become an Observation and Assessment Centre.) I was the Assistant Warden which meant being third in charge, the head of the boys' house and yet very much a basic-grade worker. Like nearly all residential workers then, I was truly resident and had a room of my own in the building. It was sandwiched between two dormitories and had a glass door with a curtain over it. The trap door for the fire escape was in one corner and outside my door was an emergency key in a glass box! There were eight professional staff and two teachers for thirty-two children and teenagers. We regularly worked about eighty hours a week and were on call every night that we were there. Compared with many other residential workers at the time, we had good conditions and were well staffed. Again I learned a lot and fast, often through the children themselves and the mistakes I made with them. This was a benevolent and at times genuinely therapeutic place with some authentic claim to be a good setting for a lot of the children, and also for young, untrained, inexperienced workers to be taught the rudiments of residential work as a serious and challenging job, not just a stepping stone to training for field social work or a fill-in job with 'kids'.

By the early 1970s I was deputy at Frogmore, a children's home in Wandsworth, run by the London Borough of Hammersmith. A large place built in 1964, previously run as two homes where children were given the slipper if they were naughty and inspected at the gate before they went off to school, it had, by the time I went to work there, a rather chaotic air. Full of long-stay children and suffering from a crisis of staff morale, it was then designated a short-stay home and began to undergo major upheavals. Over the next few years a creative and dedicated group of workers and some brilliant children and teenagers made quite a place of Frogmore. We pioneered all sorts of new and exciting work, enlisting the help of parents, working with children partly in residence and partly in their own homes, making early attempts to confront and work against the racist and sexist practice which was as much in ourselves as workers as in anyone else. We established a culture of shared responsibility and an anti-institutional lifestyle which was centred around wonderful and at times hair-raising community meetings, special child/adult relationships and a non-hierarchial organisation of work.

I was appointed head of Frogmore in 1974 and stayed for another four years before going to Bristol University to take the one-year post-qualifying advanced course which Chris Beedell had run since 1961. I was already very interested in any available theory of residential work, had done my qualifying childcare course part-time at Southwark College, and while reading fairly widely in the area I had attended short management and groupwork courses and was absorbed in the problems of organisational design and change. At Bristol I had the chance to put a lot of this experience and interest together and particularly to reflect on my six hectic years at Frogmore. With a small group of other experienced residential workers and two rather special tutors, Chris Beedell and Roger Clough, I had the opportunity to discuss, read more deeply, write and explore new areas of work. I had three engaging and very demanding placements – at an old people's home, at the Cotswold Community, and portering at the Bristol Royal Infirmary. It was a good year for me, which I still draw on. In particular, it focussed my continuing fascination with the ways organisations work (or do not), how they can be helped to work and the relationship of organisation to task.

Later I pursued this interest in organisation and team analysis by taking the two-year, part-time advanced course in consultation at the Tavistock Clinic, and then by taking a master's degree in Public Policy Studies at Bristol's School for Advanced Urban Studies.

Meanwhile, I had spent three years working independently as a consultant and trainer, a life which brought me into contact with many social services departments and agencies. Working in groups and on courses with care assistants and other residential care workers and managers, visiting and working with a wide variety of establishments, I became increasingly interested in residential work with older people.

In 1982 the London Borough of Lambeth advertised for an officer-in-charge for Inglewood, a very large but run-down home for which there were major plans for change. I knew some of the workers from Inglewood and had heard a lot about the place. I was attracted by its apparent drawbacks of size, institutionalisation and longterm neglect; it could only get better. I took the plunge, applied for and got the job.

Here was a residential establishment at the very bottom of the heap. It was in many ways the ideal setting in which to try to implement the principles which I had developed and had practised in other situations, principles which Lambeth (to its credit) had spelled out in its own policy documents, but which (to its shame) had been unable or unwilling to implement.

Some of the story of the five years I spent at Inglewood is recorded elsewhere (Burton 1988; 1989a) but my experience of residential work there and at other places (particularly Frogmore) provides the raw material and the basis of my approach as set out in this book.

Writing now, again in practice as an independent consultant, I am using my collection of notes, reports, articles, scripts of talks and diaries which I have kept very carefully since the mid-1960s when I first found myself embroiled in this fascinating and demanding work.

What drives me to write now is an ambition to set it all down – to try to write a book about residential work which will communicate new approaches, new ways of thinking about managing and *doing* the work which have not been written in this way before. My hope is that you, the reader, will find that the more analytical and theoretical material included here lives because it is founded on my constant use of my real experience, in which you may hear, feel, remember and understand your own.

John Burton

Acknowledgements

The stories, ideas, imagination, knowledge, the long hours of trying to work it out and the moments of inspiration have come with, through and from other people. I am sharing again here what I have shared in and been part of before. I have not the space to name all those with whom I have learned but they include residents, friends, colleagues, students, staff teams, my teachers, tutors and supervisors – and my own family who have given me a rough time about *not* writing this book and have tolerated and encouraged me while I have written it. I wish to acknowledge the contributions – individual and collective – of all these people and to thank them. I hope most of them will find something in these pages which they recognise and approve of. I wait, with trepidation, to hear their other comments.

The words of Chapter 8 are not mine. They relate firsthand experiences of living in residential care. I thank the various contributors to this chapter, among whom are Sylvia Ballard, Johnny B, Florence Durnell and Patricia Ryan.

Finally, I wish to single out one person on whose individual support and encouragement I have depended – a real writer, a gentle consultant, a most helpful critic – my father.

Introduction

The structure and contents of this book are based on my own experience and learning in residential work. In the Preface I have given an account of my introduction to and subsequent career in residential care, and in Chapter 1 I recount five detailed episodes from my own work. These episodes are selected to highlight the widening range of issues and dilemmas on which I concentrate in the ensuing chapters.

In Chapter 2 I start with what it feels like to begin as a residential worker, struggling to understand and manage oneself in very testing situations. I then consider (Chapter 3) the essence of what we as workers are required to do to give and receive, to work through relationships. In Chapter 4 I discuss taking on the extra responsibilities of becoming a senior worker or a manager, moving on in Chapter 5 to the helpful organisation of residential care – the building, the decoration and furniture, organising staff, routines and rules. Chapter 6 tackles questions of how organisation can also get in the way and prevent residential care from being a good experience. I discuss the roles and functions of outsiders in Chapter 7, how they can be used and what they can contribute to successful work.

For Chapter 8 I asked a range of people who live or have lived in different sorts of residential homes to talk of their experiences and ideas: what works and doesn't work; what contribution staff can and do make; how places should be organised, and many other aspects of life 'in residence'. In Chapter 9 I look at the politics of residential care and social services and I sketch out a vision for the future.

You will see from that rather stark summary of the contents that the book moves progressively from the individual worker/resident relationship, through the group, the team, the establishment, to the wider organisation and the political and social context of the work. A more comprehensive and detailed view of how the book is structured will be gained from the Contents pages on which chapter titles and subheadings are given, and from the lists of all Examples and Checklists.

I hope this book will have many uses for a wide range of readers. It is intended to be read from beginning to end! However, I know I am not the only person who rarely reads this sort of book in that way. Most parts of the book will stand on their own but will lead you on or back to other connected parts. In particular, you may find that the Examples (of which there are thirty), plus the five episodes in Chapter 1, give attractive and immediate access to your current areas of interest and concern. I envisage that these Examples (all of which are taken from real events) will be useful in teaching and training.

In the sense that it is not highly theoretical, this is not a difficult book to read. It is full of stories, and if you have any experience of the work you will recognise many of the dilemmas, struggles and rewards of the job. In another sense it may be difficult: there are a lot of questions, many of them very personal, and very few answers. If you were expecting a straightforward 'how to' book, you will be disappointed, although you will find a good deal of practical guidance throughout, often summarised in the form of Checklists. When I do offer answers of any sort, they are my own ways forward in particular situations. I don't prescribe them and I hope you don't swallow them whole.

You may also be surprised to find scant attention to subjects you may initially search for: keyworking, care plans, contracts, normalisation, team building, advocacy, complaints, quality assurance, competences, delegation. I believe if you use the book in conjunction with your own experience, ideas and aspirations you will find that all the issues underlying these subjects *are* discussed but not in the way and not from the direction to which you may be accustomed. I ask *you* to feel, and think and find your own way through. That is exactly what you have to do in the work.

I wish to be plain about my enthusiasm and idealism for residential work and through this book to set out and proclaim the arguments for its liberating power. There is clearly a need now to create and sustain fundamental change in the institutions themselves, so that instead of damaging people whom they are intended to help they can fulfil their positive potential. In spite of all the mistakes I have made, I am proud to have worked in, and now still to contribute to, some institutions which were or are, at times, truly liberating.

It is not usual to write about residential work for all user groups but my experience has been varied and I see much more which unifies, for example, work with children and work with pensioners than divides them.

Indeed, I envisage (in the face of the present stampede towards specialisation) that one of the future developments for residential centres will be to offer a wide mixture of services which are *not* defined by excluding ages or levels of handicap, or types of behaviour or definitions of disability, but include and welcome all users as active contributors to open community services centred in and reaching out from a building. (This vision is described in detail in Chapter 9.)

I want to communicate a philosophy, an approach and practice which *work*, in an area where too few of our past and present institutions have worked. The tendency now is to find an alternative mode of care; the old homes were expensive, institutionalising and ineffective, the argument goes, let's scrap them and save ourselves a lot of money and aggravation. An unhappy and unloved child in a foster home is cheaper and not half so much managerial responsibility or public liability, providing agreed procedures are exactly followed, as the same child in a children's home. An old person dying at home isn't a scandal as long as all the available services can be proved to have been 'delivered' (like the milk!), whereas the same person dying in an old people's home may raise a storm of questions about levels of care, control, staffing, medication and institutionalisation. One of the greatest barriers to good residential care is the hoary, but currently orthodox, notion that institutions are bad and cannot be a part of the community, whereas families or the 'community' are good.

If residential care remains isolated behind its walls, its unkempt municipal gardens, and its locked front doors, if the staff and residents are segregated in hierarchies and public loneliness, if all we hear about residential community living are the cruel and frightening scandals of abuse and corruption, these homes will remain weak and ineffective – to be opened and closed, run down and hived off, dominated and despised at will. However, if they work on their most basic advantage and foundation of people living and working together, creatively and cooperatively, in the real world, they can be marvellous, rich, vibrant – *and* economic, efficient and effective – places. My central objective in this book is to discuss and demonstrate, to discover and divine how the liberating potentialities of residential care can be achieved.

Chapter 1

Scenes from residential work

The five scenes from residential work described in this chapter are drawn from my own experience. I have chosen these particular events and situations because they cover a wide area and exemplify the complex and pressing demands that the work makes on us. They relate directly to all the subsequent chapters, in which the issues raised by the stories are discussed in detail.

I have ordered the stories, not chronologically, but in the same way as the book is structured, exploring first the feelings, thoughts and actions of individual workers engaged with assisting an individual resident. I then consider the building of relationships, the worker as part of a team, the resident as part of a group, questions of leadership and management, the way a whole establishment functions. The scenes broaden further to illustrate the wider political and organisational encompassments that so crucially affect residential care, ostensibly sustaining, but all too often hindering, the accomplishment of the primary task.

STRUGGLING TO CARE

Below I describe about twenty minutes of an evening's work of two staff in a large, traditionally run, old people's home. Inglewood, in the London Borough of Lambeth was reorganised over the five years since the time of this account to become a much more attractive and useful institution, with many different supportive functions, operating in smaller units, staffed by integrated teams of workers, and existing as part of a neighbourhood network of services for pensioners.

Viola and I went into room 13 where there were four beds. It was occupied by four old women who were all incontinent, two doubly. They were in their late eighties and nineties and all were what was known as 'confused', or, because of their multiple physical and mental frailties, they were often called 'the babies'. The whole of this passage (the 'babies' passage') on the ground floor smelled very strongly of urine. It had soaked into the floor coverings and the mattresses; the smell permeated the curtains, wallpaper and furniture. Sheets, blankets and clothing, although washed, were stained and had an unpleasant odour even after cleaning.

Mrs Pollard was sitting propped up in her bed. She had a strong growth of dark hair on her face and the slate-grey hair on her head lay straggly and dirty against the pillows. She had ceased to communicate with words; instead she grunted and when in obvious pain, but sometimes inexplicably, she let out a high-pitched shout or yelp. We were used to this sound from many residents as they got near to dying; nevertheless it was inhuman and frightening.

It was 7 p.m. Mrs Pollard needed changing, which had probably been done at about 2.30 p.m. before the early shift had gone off duty. We both knew what lay under the bedclothes. Mrs Pollard was wet and soiled. We needed to wash her, change her nightie, change all the sheets and possibly some blankets. But much worse than that, since she had been in bed for some weeks now, the deep and spreading sores on her body had deteriorated terribly.

She was a very heavy woman, sixteen stones, and difficult to move. She had large but superficial sore patches beneath her breasts. On her buttocks were two deep sores nearly exposing the bone (bone was visible here on another resident) and beneath the bandages on her feet, her heels were rotting sponges of stinking, dead flesh.

Under such an attack of deteriorating, poisoning sores and the respiratory infection which had confined her to bed, it was extraordinary that a very aged human being could survive. In such pain, with no visiting relatives or friends, with no diversion and nothing to look forward to, forced to exist in such utter degradation, what kept Mrs Pollard fighting to live?

As staff, I think, we all hoped she would die soon, for her sake and for ours, but she was holding on remarkably. A few of the staff loved Polly, as she had been affectionately nicknamed, and believed that they could tell her so by their actions, by sitting with her for a few seconds, holding her hand, giving her a drink from a feeding cup, stroking her face. Ellen, a domestic worker, was actually sitting with her when she eventually died.

But Mrs Pollard represented work that could never be done, a huge burden of disgust, resentment and guilt, a terrifying chasm of compassion that could not be filled and could not be crossed. Staff were left struggling with it, without help, respect or understanding, and equally undignified, reviled for being who they were in the job they had been given but could not do.

After more or less successfully washing Mrs Pollard from head to shin, changing the sheets and the pillow cases, putting cream on the sores under her breasts, trying to clean and dress the deep sores on her buttocks (we had no training or direction in how or what to use), Viola and I looked at each other.

The operation so far had taken us about twenty minutes. Viola was working fast and efficiently. I was her apprentice. She had led the way in washing, turning, the hard-learned techniques of taking off and putting on clothes, of changing bedding with someone in the bed, of removing heavily soiled sheets, of lifting a large, inert body. In between assisting in the room, I had run off searching for sheets, a nightdress, the cream, all in very short supply and from common stock. Viola carried a wash bag with her, provided by herself, without which there would not have been a flannel or soap, and which included talcum powder and a bottle of shampoo. The few residents who owned such personal items were the strong (in mind or body) who had managed to protect territory and possessions and had their own rooms, or those who had strong advocates in relatives or visiting friends. This was a small minority.

We had done everything except Mrs Pollard's heels. Two days ago a district nurse had dressed them. We knew that they needed to be dressed now; the bandages were soaked with urine and the smell of putrefaction overrode the other smells in the room even through the bandages. Two washed bandages hung on the rail of the bedside locker. When we got the old ones off we would face damage for which we had no treatment. We would do our best to clean the heels but the flesh would come away as we did it. We had nothing to put on them apart from some gauze, if we could find it in the medical room, and the washed, cleanish bandages.

There were more than a hundred residents in the home, at least half of whom would have to be helped to bed, and given some of the attention we had given to Mrs Pollard. There were three others in this room alone and altogether there were four staff working on the late shift.

Wordlessly, shamefully, Viola and I decided to do no more. We repositioned the metal cradle over Mrs Pollard's feet to stop the weight of the bedding pressing down on her heels, and carefully pulled up the sheets and blankets, tucking them in neatly around her, and after touching her hand or patting her cheek, wished her goodnight before hurrying on to the next job. The night staff would change her and perhaps dress her heels later.

Mrs Pollard died about a week after this evening, poisoned by her sores.

COMPLICATED, EXHAUSTING WORK

This story is about work with children and teenagers (and one in particular) at Frogmore, a local authority Community Home for up to thirty residents.

It is summer 1974. There is a group of children and adults in Richmond Park in southwest London. I am there, the most senior and experienced of the grown-ups (but still relatively young and inexperienced); the children and teenagers, ranging from eight to fifteen, are scrambling around and playing a game which involves being, or sighting and chasing imaginary creatures like elves – bonkazoolas, I think we called them. The game has no rules or form; you don't have to say you are playing and you can talk and walk along at the same time. This was a game that just sprang up that sunny evening, was played once or twice more in similar circumstances and faded away. Bonkazoolas were mostly friendly, interesting, shy and charming, but also very unpredictable because we never knew who was who – was I a bonkazoola or was I chasing a bonkazoola? – or whether there even were such creatures in the long grass, trees and undergrowth.

Throughout this game Lorna stayed close to me. She would jump on my back, have a piggy-back for a few yards, run off, hide, but most of the time she was having another conversation which wended its way in and out of the running and tumbling game. It was only possible to have this conversation at this stage because of the game.

She was telling me about her past. She had been born and brought up in Jamaica by her granny who had died, and then she had joined her mother on a huge and soulless old council estate in west London. There are very few children in this predicament now but in the 1960s and early 1970s this was a common situation and one I was used to (as a childcare worker). Many women of Lorna's age now are bringing up their own Black British children. Although I was familiar with the situation and I had tried to imagine what it would be like, I could never get very close to a deep understanding of the effects of such a huge separation, loss and the shock of arriving in a White, racist society to a new mother.

This had all happened in the previous year for Lorna. She was thirteen. This precarious mother/daughter relationship fell apart very quickly under the pressure of school, friends, being out and about in this empty, unwholesome, urban environment. Her mother couldn't control her; Lorna didn't respond to the chastisement and her mother began to be frightened of her, convinced at one time that her daughter was trying to poison her.

The situation came to such a head that she came very willingly in to local authority care a few days before the evening I am describing. At that time all of the staff at Frogmore, the children's home she first came to, were

> White, and probably slightly more than half the children were Black, mostly
> Afro-Caribbean, though that wasn't a phrase in common usage.

The term Afro-Caribbean is now itself beginning to be dropped, as a much
larger proportion of this population of the United Kingdom were born or
have spent most of their lives in Britain. A Black (African) person with a
Caribbean heritage may in a few years time be more likely to describe her
or himself as African British (or English, Irish, Scots or Welsh), a British
person of African descent, or an African person of British nationality and
citizenship. However, such progress is a long struggle and will require a
pride and appreciation from British people (particularly White) in living
in a multiracial society. This issue has a strong influence on the effectiveness and quality of all residential care.

Officially, even in this comparatively progressive local authority, there
was no substantial recognition that the needs of Black children in care
were essentially any different from those of White children, nor was there
any great concern that an all-White staff group was unsuitable to do a good
job for Black children.

> So there was Lorna establishing what can be seen as a therapeutic relation-
> ship with a White male worker and at the same time telling him in the most
> influential way that he had yet heard about the experience of loss, separ-
> ation, rejection, cultural and racial disconnection and the severance of
> family ties – and many other things besides. And all this in the middle of a
> complicated and engaging game being played on and off by about a dozen
> people at one corner of Richmond Park.

The development of, what I call here, a therapeutic relationship is in many
ways chancey and haphazard. There may be a fortunate context which just
happens to be right, as on that particular evening. Mistakes are frequent
but often become significant parts of the relationship; their destructive
threat can be overcome, made constructive and integrated. The frightening
but so productive content of transference and counter-transference (see
Chapter 3) are used most often quite unwittingly. (Sometimes, if you knew
what was happening, you would run a mile!) What parent/child link and
communication was going on? Who was initiating it? Was there a sexual
meaning to this horseplay? Was this closeness and touch legitimate? Was
this girl – this man – safe?

There is no time to debate, even mentally question, your actions and attitudes. You think about them afterwards and if you are lucky in residential work, you have someone to talk to about them (through supervision, support, staff meetings and staff groupwork). But, working well, there are mechanisms of test and control and awareness, which are taking stock, guiding and keeping one tiny important element of your consciousness on the outside looking in. The mistakes are made when these mechanisms (part of you) cannot keep up or are confused by the multiplicity of events and emotions.

> It was a beautiful, sunny evening and that rambling, tumbling group of children and adults were happy and unusually collected in their behaviour. (This was demonstrated by their capacity to enjoy and tolerate such a loose and anarchic game.) There was a rare lack of aggression and I was more relaxed than I often was in such situations. More usually I would be sharply aware of and anxious about the potential chaos in which many of the children we worked with found their most self-destructive, frightened but habitual behaviour.

To go back to the previous and very different evening: we are still with Lorna although this story involves many other people. The following is the exact diary account I wrote at the time; it is therefore not necessarily expressed precisely as I would like to write it now.

> *Before tea* Allan and Django were caught on top of a lorry belonging to the packing yard which gives us wood. A tarpaulin has been torn and other damage done to crates. It is not certain whether or not Allan and Django actually caused this damage. I saw Allan first and took him to the office where I questioned him and 'told him off'.
>
> Soon after tea as we were just going to cricket, I saw Allan outside the gates, called to him, but he ran off and although I gave chase he eluded me.
>
> *Cricket* When we eventually turned up at the park, we started reasonably promptly but Terry was not picked on my side. He was now 'in a mood'. This was made ten times worse when he was out first ball! for which he seemed to blame me although I had no hand in his dismissal. He then stalked around for a while before, towards the end of his side's innings, picking up the ball and hiding it so that we could not continue with the game. We finally got the ball back from him only to be again frustrated by Fred's getting it and holding up the game once more. I asked him to return it several times

without results. I got angry with Fred (mistake), grabbed him and took the ball. Fred said I'd hurt him and 'made him angry now' and began to head for home. I went after him and said he couldn't go, but would have to field or sit and watch. (His side was now fielding.) I held on to him and he struggled and shouted and threatened until it was my turn to bat and I had to leave him in order not to completely wreck the game. He went back to Frogmore. (See Mike's notes about the evening.)

11– and 12–year-olds' meeting We started this as soon as we returned from the cricket in order not to lose the conversation which was already taking place, i.e. whether I was right or wrong to physically hold Fred. There was a strong feeling that I was bullying and unfair, that I had no right to 'order' children around – 'You can't tell us what to do.' We went on about staff, violence, and violence between children for a long time. Terry was still furious and resentful to me even at the end of the meeting. Karl made some penetrating and mature comments. Geoff was his usual benign, foggy self.

Pauline and Lorna persistently interrupted the meeting for about twenty minutes.

13-, 14– and 15–year-olds' meeting At first it seemed that no-one would come to the meeting. Dan, Chrissie and Kate turned up. Then Desmond and Shirley came in and just hung on. We began falteringly but quite amicably. We had coffee.

Pauline and Lorna stormed in, all wet from paddling in puddles and raving in the rain. They were full of 'going to a club' earlier on; they weren't coming to the meeting. Pauline was changing her mind all the time; she'd never asked for a meeting etc. But they stayed. Both in a very high mood. Shouting, anti Chrissie and Kate. Eventually we got onto childhood – first memories. This became quite fruitful and Lorna pretended she was a baby, and much to everyone's amusement and intense interest, cried and kicked on the floor. Most of the children were a little apprehensive of the idea of searching back to their childhoods and were reticent, perhaps using Lorna's outrageous and forthright exhibition as a substitute for their own memories. It provoked great outbursts of laughter.

Julie's visit (Steve's mother) Towards the end of the adolescents' meeting, Pauline had gone out and returned with the news that there was a mad, drunk woman outside. Lorna was out of the door in a flash followed by some others. Reluctant to leave the meeting on any pretext, but sensing some serious situation, I followed them and left Pete [staff] to finish off the meeting. On the front lawn stood a swaying, bellowing, blaspheming woman with a crowd of children from the flats leaning over the wall jeering and goading her. Immediately she saw me she came at me and grabbed me by the arms, and started to shout threats at me. I soothed her and told her I would protect her, and she was safe (great stuff!), and she gradually quietened. Anne ([resident] brought a cigarette for her and she began to move where I was pushing her gently away from the children at the wall. All this time Lorna was darting in and out very like a little dog, yelping hysterically, and the children at the wall were hurling abuse and shouting out 'Steve hanged himself!' (which he apparently tried to do). Julie (the woman, who lives in the next block of flats) wanted to telephone Steve, her son, so I took her first to the front house and tried to make the call for her but could not get the 2p in! (Steve is at the moment in a Classifying School which Julie refers to kindly as a 'mental home'.) My original aim had been to try to just get her home but the children outside wouldn't move away and I couldn't get her through them.

Before failing at the front house phone, I managed to communicate to Linda [staff] that a surreptitious call to the police might be useful since the situation still looked potentially very nasty. Julie and I went to the office to phone Steve and she calmed down a bit more. Before we got into the office, Lorna came to me and very urgently, almost desperately but quietly said, 'Get her out of here.' In the office we got through to Steve, and Julie talked to him for ages. The police came in very tactfully, and eventually Julie left with them happy to go home, and all was O. K. ... not quite all because...

Lorna – bedtime After all this excitement, Lorna was pretty high and was prancing around with an umbrella. It was way past her bedtime and I walked down to the gate to chat a bit while I slowly told her that it *was* time for bed and that she *should* be going. After a few minutes we went in but immediately re-emerged when she spotted three boys talking to Pauline at the gate. The presence of the boys made her show off, parading up and down, and refusing to get ready. I went on telling her and then said quite finally that she *had to* go to bed. She ran up the road when I moved towards her; I followed. She, willing to be 'caught', let me lift her cradled in my arms, and when that was too tiring I carried her piggy-back.

As soon as we got inside the front door, she began to create mayhem. I told her she had to sit calmly for ten minutes by my watch before she went to prepare for bed. She screamed and hollered, as I took her firmly by the arm to the playroom. Each time she made for the door I brought her back. [The playroom had glass doors so we were in full view of other children and staff passing by and looking in curiously.] I talked most of the time, keeping a running commentary going. Sometimes she sat on the floor, sometimes leant by the wall. We talked a lot between screaming sessions, carrying on with the main theme of the meeting, childhood memories – her granny, her mother, coming to London, etc.

Eventually she agreed to start ten minutes calm, and she did very well and went up. But once upstairs she began to laugh loudly and after warning her once, I brought her down again and told her she had to sit quietly for half an hour before I would be convinced that she was ready to go upstairs.

We went through a few minutes of screaming and then started the half hour, but this time there was no talk. She was tired and a bit tearful. She went up when it was time and went quietly to bed – but did give me her trousers which she had washed, for me to put in the drier to be ready for school tomorrow.

Looking back now, I am amazed by our faith and energy. The account is littered with glaring mistakes, events which I would handle differently now and record differently, but the overwhelming impression as I recollect the situation is of how a group of us continued to struggle to establish good, consistent, therapeutic work out of the most adverse conditions. It is difficult now to appreciate the pace, the physical and emotional strain of the work, or to comprehend the formidable problems of managing such an establishment in a way that eventually truly engaged and made concrete progress with very troubled children and adolescents, with race and gender issues for staff, children and families, and with the non-hierarchical and self-managing running of the home. I have no doubt that this is the situation which still faces workers who have a longterm view, and intend to try to put principle in practice.

Another more specific and painful recollection is also at the forefront of my memory: our use of physical holding of children (which nowadays always seems to be called restraint) when we did not know and could not manage any other way of getting some control. I can recall the absolute necessity of establishing some order being so often uppermost in my mind and my instincts at the time. We had eschewed many of the formal structures, routines and punishments which had themselves been utterly unsuited to the task of providing for these children. Those previous forms of control (many impersonally violent themselves) had repeatedly failed. The children's resistance to institutional order and punishment had in itself become a living culture – a subculture – which distracted from the painful, destructive, emotional turmoil in which many of the children lived. However, in order to grapple with such turmoil and to make any progress in creating a calmer and more therapeutic environment, we found ourselves as workers initially – sometimes ridiculously, sometimes violently and occasionally entirely appropriately – grappling with the children themselves. Some of this violence was not of our or the children's making, but was inherent in the situations we were expected to manage – ones which were often quite beyond our energy, skills and resources. Later, as we learned to manage and resist unreasonable outside pressures and to identify, for instance, gender-specific elements of violent situations, we reduced violent incidents dramatically (Senior 1989).

ARGUING WITH BERTRAM

This story is set in Inglewood again, the old people's home, a couple of years later than the first story about Mrs Pollard. I was doing much less direct work with users than I did at Frogmore, but the population of residents and staff was much larger – about 150 people. The internal and external organisational complexities and pressures were much greater, and we were working in a much more public and politically volatile arena.

Here again let me describe to you an encounter with just one person and move from this into the context of the whole place. This account is not from the establishment's log book but is written from my own detailed notes made at the time.

I crouch by Bertram's bed. It is about 11 p.m. and I should have been off duty (but on call) for an hour. In fact I have been having my usual meeting with the night staff and have just walked around downstairs checking doors and windows in the passages, staircases and public rooms. The building is very insecure and subject to break-ins; and like every other building of its type and use it is also particularly vulnerable to fire. In fact this is what the night staff and I have been discussing, with special reference to Bertram who is very fond of candles, and claims that one of his jobs in the place is 'fireman'.

I have gone in ostensibly to say goodnight to Bertram but really to do what I can to ensure that he is not lighting a little fire on a tin tray in the middle of his room or has not lit candles on his windowsill. (He has done both several times over the past few weeks.) Bertram's enthusiasms go in phases. Just as his fireman's duties seem to include lighting fires, so later do his 'security guard' duties include going out in the middle of the night, leaving outside doors unlocked.

He is an unusual, charming and interesting man who, in spite of his evident mental illness and at times very aggressive behaviour, is loved and respected by most of the staff.

When the electricity was cut off in his council flat, he took up the floor boards to burn to keep himself warm. Significantly, his trade was a floorer. He is a person of contradictions and spirit. After we have known him for quite a long time, we learn that his stories of a wife and son both in long-stay hospitals are true and he has a great concern for them.

He is not old by the standards of most of his fellow residents. Remarkably, he has managed to hold on to his pension book and rarely pays his bill to the local authority. He knows that they are more or less powerless to force him to pay up and, as staff, some of us are rather pleased that he and the one or two other residents (who though they do pay regularly have still retained their books) have succeeded in resisting the disgraceful institutional domination represented by the appropriation of pension books by the council [a process which they have condemned in policy but continue in practice].

I knock on the door of room 7. Bertram bids me enter and I find him lying as usual on the steel-sprung base of his bed (he didn't believe in mattresses at this time) with a lighted candle on his bedside cupboard.

I, tired and desperate to get away from any further complications of the evening's shift, explode in anger. I open the way for this anger by telling myself that it is about time I try 'heavy' tactics with Bertram, that I have every right to be furious, and that my verbal onslaught is for everyone whose lives, jobs and wellbeing are threatened by his dangerous and arrogant actions. Voice raised in righteous indignation, I snuff the candle, pick it up and search the bare but very messy room for any others, saying, 'I don't care what you have to say or what your ridiculous arguments are for lighting candles and fires (I've heard them all before). I'm taking these away and from now on I'll come into your room whether you give me permission or not – and even if you're not here – to check that you've got no candles or other dangerous things in here.'

The room has been newly decorated only a few weeks before but Bertram removed the wash basin and the panelling around it which concealed the plumbing. He has installed precarious shelves and as I search through them I come across many familiar, long-lost objects from all over the building.

My anger boils, as all the warnings and wise words from colleagues ring in my ears: 'Bertram's got it. It's dangerous to let him lock his door. We can't go on letting him live here. Stop him.' Some of us defended: 'You can't blame Bertram for everything. He doesn't steal things, he just borrows. If we don't cope with him who will? He'll just be locked up again.' 'It's all very well for you to be understanding but you're risking other people's lives.' This debate was taking place in a home where a fire three years before *had* killed someone and had been a deeply disturbing and frightening experience for some of the staff who were involved and all the residents who were living there at the time.

I had been in this sort of position many times before with children and teenagers, but not with a pensioner. After five minutes of ranting and searching and commenting on everything I found, I walked out, sharply pulling the door closed behind me by hooking my foot round it, my arms full of a collection of jugs, candles, stationery, food, medical equipment, clothes and assorted junk.

Ten minutes later I was back crouching at Bertram's bedside trying to get across the urgency and danger of the situation, trying to apologise for my unreasonable and senseless outburst, begging Bertram to be cooperative but yet again beginning to boil with rage as all my words were steadfastly ignored, and as I felt sorry for myself and outraged by the situation that Bertram's behaviour was putting into sharp and painful focus.

I was borne down on by that huge burden of responsibility and injustice which residential workers habitually feel, and which so often hinders their work. For me that night the heavy mass of resentment went something like this:

> *Here I am responsible for this whole place, for people's lives, for well over fifty workers, for a large, crumbling unsuitable building, for managing all this and trying to change it and make it work well, with all and sundry telling me how to do it, badgering me with requests at every hour of every day, expecting me to give them support and leadership, and after a hard day when I have got to try to sleep in the bloody place, with another very hard day tomorrow, and with central management on my back all the time, jealous, critical and obstructive, but never giving me much appreciation, encouragement or support.... yes, here I am late at night with lots still to do before I can get up to that inhospitable, noisy sleeping-in room, shouting at Bertram and losing the last bit of self-respect I've got in the way of professional practice and venting my anger on someone I am not really angry with. I am tired, lonely and unhappy, and failing at the very centre of the task of a residential worker – making and maintaining constructive relationships.*

Is is at points such as this when terrible mistakes can be made and when talented workers decide to leave the job.

I was in the middle of and leading such major change at the time that I refused to let the content of these very angry feelings surface; I felt I had no-one to talk to about them and that I had to survive and cope, or else the whole hazardous project would come crashing down around us.

This leads me on to two more scenes, again about ten years apart, first at Frogmore and then at Inglewood, in which the responsibility of managing *and* being closely involved in the day to day work of a home are even more sharply in focus and conflict. I am not suggesting that the two should ever be completely separate for any member of staff or for the users; indeed, a central theme of this book is how 'doing' and 'managing' are complementary roles. My first three stories of residential work may have shown how the roles are painfully and sometimes happily joined.

My next two highlight more specifically the conflicts inherent in residential work management. Such conflicts are evident in this way only if senior workers accept active parts in direct work, administration and creative management and are trying to integrate those functions for themselves and with all users and workers in the place.

PREPARING TEA

It is about 4.30 p.m. and I am standing at a large double sink looking out of the kitchen window to the front garden, and peeling carrots. The garden is quite pretty this year. In just a small patch we have sunflowers and roses, flowering shrubs, and little pockets of annuals sown in the spring. The lawn is unusually neat and for once there isn't paper blowing around all over it. All of the plants and the state of the garden in general have specific connections with individual people, children and adults. At the back one of the older boys has built a pond. We have even made window boxes out of the wooden frames of old bed bases. The garden signifies a stage of development for the place and for many individual children, and indeed for some of us workers. Passers-by stop and look at our garden, a little oasis in the middle of a very bleak and run-down 1930s tenement estate. Even the local teenagers who sit on the front wall in the summer evenings, admire it and have shown unusual care and appreciation for it. The garden certainly says something.

With me in the kitchen, Michelle and Sandra are also engaged with getting tea ready for 6 o'clock. We are cooking for twenty-six and it's important that the meal is ready on time. At 3 p.m. four of us, the late shift of workers, sat around the kitchen table and planned our work for the evening: who was cooking tea, who would collect the children from school, who was going out that evening, what was on TV, what activities were taking place and who was seeing which children to bed.

Peter was what we called the 'duty person; – the coordinator for the day; he was in charge. That duty was formally rostered; being cook was less formal but nonetheless everyone was expected to take her or his turn; it was, after all, one of the most crucial jobs in the place. It also involved the residents, both cooking and eating. Sometimes older children would be in charge in the kitchen with a member of staff assisting them. Two other colleagues were, by 4.30, just returning from the school run, picking up children who for some reason couldn't or shouldn't make it back to Frogmore on their own from their various schools. They were also picking up Michelle's mother who was coming for tea and to stay for the evening.

This was already a complicated scene to keep in my head as I stood at the sink peeling those carrots. The radio was playing the station which Michelle and Sandra had wanted, not the one I wanted, although I had managed to negotiate a reduction in volume. We talked over the top of it.

As I looked out at the garden, beginning to enjoy my evening's work, I saw Martin, a fifteen-year-old boy who was having extreme school and family difficulties. He looked like thunder. He pushed open the heavy metal gate, banging it back against the brick wall, and walked straight across the garden, trampling plants on his way to the front door.

'Martin!' I shouted about the plants, upset that our garden had to suffer because something had happened to disturb Martin. But then I controlled my first impulse which was to go and confront him about the garden; his mood had nothing to do with the garden or me yet. What Martin needed was comfort, understanding, perhaps guidance about the issue – whatever it was, an airing of feelings not just an acting out of them; not, as he was rapidly setting up, a flaming row about some trampled plants, however significant and precious they were to the rest of us. Martin was trying to take as many people as possible with him chasing a red herring. He wanted the obliterating and self-justifying power of a row; he had frequent rows with nearly everyone about apparently insignificant things.

So this time, I didn't engage with Martin straightaway. He had ignored my shout in any case and I was not the best person to offer him understanding; we had too long a history of controlling confrontation. I rang Peter from the extension in the kitchen to alert him to the situation.

Peter was in the office, getting money from the safe for one of the children. All of us, even the duty person, usually kept away from the office at times when most of the children were around, except to get things such as keys, letters or money which the children needed. Most outsiders had learned that calls should be concentrated between nine in the morning and three in the afternoon. However, as soon as I had spoken to Peter about Martin, the phone rang again in the office. The assistant director was calling to discuss a particularly problematic admission.

We had been negotiating for some months about trying to establish clearer criteria for accepting children at Frogmore, and an upper limit to what we could manage in the way of a workload. In many ways this had been going on for years without being resolved. While the building could physically hold thirty-one residents, this had long been an impractical number and twenty-two was being accepted as a 'maximum accommodation figure'. However, the least onerous task was *accommodating* children, and of course the work and time which children needed varied according to their circumstances. For instance, at the most basic level, we had found that children who weren't at school must be given full and proper attention, including organising educational work for them, during the school day. This required planning staff time.

The assistant director was now phoning himself to tell us that we had to take a very demanding thirteen-year-old boy who was not on a school roll and would need considerable but currently unavailable staff resources. We had already said that we were not in a position to accept the boy; we were already working with several children who were equally or more demanding, and our work with them would be harmed by overloading us.

After a lengthy conversation with Peter, and getting no further, the assistant director demanded that he spoke with me as the manager of Frogmore. [My awful official title then was 'superintendent'.] Although it was explained that I was cooking tea and probably doing half a dozen other things at the same time, he still insisted that I spoke to him.

We were in the middle of one of those periods in the day of a children's home when all available staff resources [in this instance, four people] should be concentrated on being alert to and meeting the needs of children returning from what for most of them was a considerable challenge – the school day.

So I was peeling the carrots; the school run had returned; there were disturbing noises overhead in the bedrooms above the kitchen; children were coming to the kitchen door and some coming in for milk or a snack. Martin was somewhere in the house, probably not being attended to and looking for a distracting row to have with someone; we had an anxious and hesitant parent for tea; my two co-cooks were asking me about the quantity of rice for twenty-six, and the kitchen extension rang with the assistant director of social services telling me that we had to accept this boy, but pretending that he was discussing the issues with me.

There was a serious gap of understanding and experience here! How could I describe to this man the scene of which I was part, which encapsulated the very reasons why we were not able to accept the boy he was trying to force in. He didn't understand, first, why Peter had so strongly resisted his demand that he should speak to me, second, what cooking the tea actually entailed in such an establishment (why didn't we get a cook?) and, third, what on earth I was doing in the kitchen and what Peter, a relatively junior member of staff, was doing in the office and in charge of the place that evening. Surely it was axiomatic that the head should have been doing that duty – 'Isn't that what we appoint superintendents for?'

It was not as if we hadn't tried to explain or had not formally set out the method of work which we employed. Our method had achieved some success, especially when compared with the other homes in the borough, and it was because of that success that we were under pressure to take this particular boy, whom it was thought other homes could not work with or, as the official terminology has it, 'contain'.

Much later that evening I drafted a long and detailed letter to the assistant director spelling out our current workload, asking for a more consistent method of resolving this issue of admissions, and giving him as much information as possible. At the end of the letter I invited him to make a decision in the light of all the circumstances, including my statement that much of the substantial progress we were making with the children we were currently working with and the longterm well-being of the home itself were in serious jeopardy.

Bob, the child in question, did not come and some progress, albeit merely temporary, was made towards a more thoughtful and efficient system of establishing suitable upper limits to our workload.

Although the assistant director's approach at the time seemed ignorant and insensitive, and was experienced as undermining and even aggressive, such effects were neither deliberate nor desired on his part. Like most managers in social services, even those who are specialist managers of residential work, he had little knowledge of the implications of what he was asking or of the nature of the work that we were doing.

However, such managers need to learn more about what it is they are managing. (They are, I hope, part of my readership.) Their job, after all, is to support and encourage what is a good and effective service, to allow such work to flourish, but to be able to distinguish it from the poor and ineffective which they much help to change. But if they do the opposite, as does unfortunately, and commonly happen, they actively and destructively interfere with the more useful but challenging establishments while tolerating and indulging those places which give very little trouble and even less real service.

LOCAL POLITICS

My last story in this chapter is set at Inglewood in the mid-1980s. With it we move one step further into the environment of residential care services – local politics. Whether private, voluntary or local authority, all residential homes exist within a political environment. but a local authority home has the most direct connections and dependency on the local council.

After creating smaller living units with their own dining rooms and kitchens at Inglewood, we began to develop the dining hall for day centre and other uses. For a few months it was used very successfully by a centre for people with severe learning disabilities whose own premises needed emergency building work. Stimulated by this experience we were discussing the possibility of creating day centre facilities which could take in younger people with disabilities as well as older people. The original plan had been to establish a centre (for social support, education and cultural events) and luncheon club for pensioners, and to use the dining hall, kitchens, toilets and a couple of rooms nearby for major social and other events. The residents of the building had a strong interest in how the space was to be used, and local people and organisations were also interested. All these people were involved in the planning process. Day care and luncheon club members had begun to use the hall, which was also in frequent use for social events.

Lambeth, the council we were working within, was, with Liverpool, at the forefront of local government opposition to the Conservative government's attempts to cut public spending and to weaken, then conquer left wing Labour councils. The council was rate capped and the Labour majority were being threatened with being barred from office for overspending and failing to set a rate. [Later they were barred from office.] The council had a lot of public support for its attempt to 'protect jobs and services'.

Behind the scenes however, there was much in-fighting and political rivalry. Chairs and vice-chairs of committees fought each other for ascendency. There were camps and factions. From the inside the services and practice didn't look so 'well worth defending' [a council slogan of the time] as they should have done.

The social services committee had been put under sustained pressure from parents and carers of people with learning disabilities to provide sufficient care services. The council increasingly made promises which they could not keep. With the temporary use of Inglewood's old dining hall by the centre for people with learning disabilities, someone got the bright idea that a total takeover of the whole of that part of the building, and permanent conversion to a new (and separate) use, would be a relatively quick, cheap and simple way of making good some of the broken promises.

In no time at all, a plan was concocted and put to the social services committee. There was considerable opposition at the committee meeting from residents and staff of Inglewood and from the parents and carers of the disabled people, who considered the solution quite unsuitable. Both groups joined forces to lobby the meeting, and managers and councillors were shocked and angry to see senior citizens, moreover residents of one of 'their' old people's homes, participating in this assertive fashion in their political process. [The more detailed story of that event is told elsewhere: Burton 1989b.]

Soon after this meeting we received notice that the social services committee would be meeting 'on site' (which meant in the dining hall!) and would the kitchen prepare drinks and food for the councillors and officers who would be there. Neither residents nor staff were invited. The refreshments which were specified were not usually provided for residents nor were the catering staff able to prepare them without taking some time away from their normal business of getting lunch ready for residents.

At first I just felt like saying, 'No. Unless you can arrange it properly and with respect for residents and staff, we'll just shut the doors.' But having thought about it and taken wise counsel with tenants [which is how we referred to residents] and colleagues, I realised that such action would only provoke a further onslaught. [There was a lot of talk of closures at the time.] However, we did decide that we would attend the meeting, though uninvited, on the grounds that the committee would need to hear our points of view in order to make their decision.

A group of tenants and staff discussed how we would handle making our representations and we predicted that the tenants would have a more powerful message to give than staff. Also they would be very difficult to shut up! Two residents were chosen to lead our side of the debate and they prepared what they intended to say.

When the committee arrived we welcomed them politely and, much to the embarrassment of some of the senior managers, stated our intention to speak to the meeting and then to leave them to get on with their business. I, as the manager of Inglewood, was introduced to the chair of the committee, who, instead of saying, 'hello' and asking about the home and what was happening there, simply said to me, 'Yes, I've heard about you. I can assure you that if senior managers can't manage you, I will.' and turned away.

When the meeting started, the two tenants spoke up wonderfully – with power and passion. We could see the committee members were stunned by the realisation that there was such a process as democracy and they had just been on the receiving end of it from people whom they regarded as too old, and infirm in mind and body to be able to take part in making decisions about their home. We all, residents and staff, left the meeting.

We were never told what exactly occurred after we had left but the chair appeared to be very upset about the outcome. On her way out, she tore down pictures and posters. She even ripped a notice off the front door which told visitors what bell to ring at night when the front doors were locked!

The old dining room was not commandeered and the new centre for people with learning disabilities was set up elsewhere.

When residential establishments are run by large organisations there is always an inherent tension between on one side the residents, their relations and friends and the staff, and on the other side policy and decision makers outside the homes. Part of the work of staff is to continuously encourage and support residents in taking power and exercising it. Some of this power will be held by staff in the home, some by outsiders like senior managers and councillors. To accomplish this transfer of power, staff have to practise a mixture of seemingly contradictory behaviours – stepping forward and stepping back, taking initiative and letting it go, protesting, demanding, asserting but then accepting, conciliating and compromising. But the process amounts to *letting go of power*. These ways of behaving are primarily geared to the advancement of residents' wellbeing and that of the residential home as a whole, but they are incomprehensible and mystifying to too many managers and councillors, who despite their proclaimed adherence to professional and/or political principle, are preoccupied with personal ambition and the consolidation of their own power.

Chapter 2

Understanding and managing
Making a start

STARTING WORK

Every reader knows what it is like to start in a new job, or a course, or to be in any strange situation with other people, not knowing what exactly is going on or what you are expected to do. In these circumstances we employ considerable emotional energy trying to understand and manage – ourselves.

In a residential work setting the feelings of confusion, anxiety and apprehension are especially intense. In my preface I tell the story of my introduction to a probation hostel: I hadn't a clue what was going on and I was struggling to manage myself for survival. A teacher facing a class for the first time in a school is subject to some of the same anxieties, although in most school settings the roles and rules of the engagement are more clearly understood by all concerned. Imagine a residential worker arriving on her first day, or even visiting an establishment prior to being interviewed, and being confronted by a child climbing in through the window of the room in which she is sitting, or by an adult crying out, 'Please help me'. What does she do? How far does she go with the remonstration about the window, or when she realises that the person who is asking for help and who clearly needs help, cannot or will not say what the problem is? What does our new worker do about the toilet door which is left open with someone sitting on the lavatory, or what does she say to the member of staff who asks her, 'Have you worked with these before?' meaning this 'sort' of client? What would you do?

Managing yourself

Immediately there are pressures put on you to behave in many different ways: do you collude? do you confront? do you run for help or ask what the rules are? do you withdraw? Everything you have been told about the place and the way it works is forgotten or simply not evident in the situations before you.

The one thing uppermost in your mind is to *survive*. The responses you make this first day will be with you long afterwards. And in struggling to survive you may behave in ways you hoped you would not.

Your most essential and reliable support will be your *self* and what you know about yourself. Your struggle will be to understand and manage yourself in this situation. What resources in you can you draw on? Your ideas, beliefs and principles – the ones you brought with you to the job, and which may have played a large part in your application and your selection for the job. Your ability to be aware of how you are feeling and to express that with some confidence, knowing it and believing it to be important. Your courage in acting authentically – being true to yourself. And later, you may learn and develop for yourself a range of practical skills of self-management.

As you respond, engage and act – you work. The child was expecting a response from you when he climbed through the window: he may well have come in through the door had you not been there! The person crying out, 'Please help me' was calling to you, although she may plead for help constantly, irrespective of whether a member of staff is there or not. As you note your own inner responses and attempt to act on them, you may also be trying to understand what this resident is communicating and where it is coming from in herself.

Your job now is to help to change the situation with the resident. I will be examining building and using relationships in more detail in the next chapter; in this chapter I am focussing on the understanding and management of ourselves as an essential first ingredient of doing the work. (Managing other people and a service is the subject of Chapter 4.) Workers at all levels in residential homes must learn to manage themselves in order to become the kind of people who can enable users to practise self-management. And managers outside the home must cultivate the same skills (basic skills of management) in order to give a supportive and developmental management service to residential staff.

Everyday management

The act of managing is part of everyone's life, paid and unpaid, at work and at home, even sometimes on holiday. Children do it; older people do it; we watch babies growing to do it with bodily functions, with co-ordination, speech, and emotions – with them*selves*. We call this 'child development'. Disabled people do it. It is revealing to note that 'manage' is a word that is frequently used for the extra organisation which disabled people have to perform in order to overcome handicap: 'Can you manage the stairs?', 'How did you manage the journey?' Managing is what housekeepers, family carers, group caterers, child rearers, home makers, household organisers – in other words most women (mostly) do most of their lives, unpaid. (Even writers do it – with difficulty!)

The concept of management has got quite out of hand since it became synonymous with what men do when they wear suits, become bosses and get paid more than other people for doing it. We are concerned about whether someone is a real manager or just a foreperson or supervisor. Management is defined exclusively in terms of managing other people, and its status is usually derived from counting up the number of people managed and the size of the budget.

If we look at our managers in social services, are they not often those who have least experience and knowledge of the everyday, real management issues and problems? They are mostly White men who have had to learn their brand of management from people like themselves, either on the job or on management courses. They usually know little of the complexities of running a household, or bringing up children, or caring for other dependants. Indeed for most of their lives most of them have been happily dependent themselves. All their physical and emotional needs have been catered for by other people; their food, clothes, even their leisure and social life have been arranged and organised and produced, so they can go out and, in the case of residential work, 'manage' exactly the same services for other people. This is a major contradiction.

However, the very concept of self-management implies and demands that each and every worker, individually and collectively, begins to take more responsibility – first for themselves.

Encouraging and supporting residents in making changes to their lives requires a partnership between workers and users in which power and responsibility grow through exchange and through increased self-awareness and understanding. The worker will be in the position of using her or his *self* in this transaction.

If the worker has scant personal power, or self-awareness, and if she is not able to manage her self, she will simply appear to the user as an operative, an administrator, a servant of a system, and she, as herself, will be irrelevant to the user's needs; she may be ignored, used, abused or attacked.

This essential management of self is most crucial in residential settings where much of the exchange and transaction between workers and users takes place in situations which are personally exposed and where self is so evident. There is no hiding behind a desk, a file, a telephone or correspondence; the bulk of the work does not go on in interviews, or conferences, or even home visits. Residential work takes place in the kitchen, the dining room, in front of the TV, in the bathroom, the lavatory, the bedroom, standing by the back door, or in a shop or on a bus.

To work in this fashion requires above all the constant practice of and attention to the management of self. It requires, in particular, men to learn to understand and use their selves, and to learn from what we might now term here 'women's management', to learn to relate feeling and thinking, to learn not to separate managing and doing into distinct and essentially hierarchical functions. It requires women to grasp, cultivate and promote their own practice of management and to resist incorporation into male, hierarchical and competitive management modes which, in residential work especially, are so clearly destructive and unhelpful to users.

Effective residential workers are constantly tuned in to what is happening inside themselves and using that awareness to manage their work. They recognise and value creativity, emotionality, sexuality and spirituality as their fundamental resources for doing the job and they use these continuously as the bases for managing their interaction with the world around them.

Ways to start understanding and managing

Ideally, you would be helped to tune in and then to utilise and translate this awareness into working resources through supervision (Chapter 5, Supervision, p. 105). But, whether you have access to regular supervision or not, some of this work will be done by you alone. Partly it will be done in solitary, quiet thinking and reflecting time and partly it will happen as you are engaged with the situations you are managing.

First I list some questions you may ask yourself about self-awareness, about your own experience, emotional maturity, ability to understand yourself and what makes you tick – the elements of your own make-up which would enable you to work in a setting where the strongest of emotional demands will be made on you. These are questions to ponder and explore and of course, if possible, to discuss in supervision; they are not questions with yes or no answers!

Understanding yourself in this job

* What is your experience of working with the user group?
* Are you sufficiently aware of your own involvement, responses and reactions to users in direct work to then work with colleagues who are undergoing similar stress and bewilderment with their own firsthand work?
* Do you have ideas about what is going on in 'therapeutic' relationships? Chapter 3 expands on this topic.
* Does your own experience help you to stumble through the maze of emotional upsets, byways, dead ends and revelations to end up making some (albeit temporary) sense of what may be going on?
* What meaning and emotional implications do the following have for you: separation, loss, death, early childhood deprivation, sexual abuse, love, hate, revulsion and attraction, depression and elation, disability, disease, divorce, racism, sexism, homophobia, ageing, institutionalisation, poverty, soiling, incontinence, sickness, aggression, drunkenness, drugs, despair and suicide? Are they simply to be 'managed' or are they real parts of real people's lives, including your own and colleagues?
* What are you feeling, allowing yourself to feel, as you read through this list? What images and memories are evoked?
* Do you try to fit this human condition and behaviour into a system, to organise them away, or can you feel them first, then think about them and finally try to build and maintain an organisation which accepts them as real and recognises their existence for people? Such an organisation's purpose is to accept the person and to work to eliminate some of those conditions and enhance and strengthen others.

Having worked on your feeling responses and increased your awareness of what is going on inside, how do you apply this to managing your work? Whether you have applied for your job and got it, or you have held the post for some months or years, you need to be clear about what the job is and what you intend to do in it.

Understanding the job

* What is your job description?
* What of the many tasks outlined can you realistically accomplish? Are there items which you need to question, even renegotiate, or (with discussion) accept cannot be done?
* What do you do for which clients?
* What to you plan to do for which clients?
* Which clients do you find yourself avoiding?
* Which clients are you most frequently with?
* Which clients provoke the strongest feelings in you?
* Do you need to train, or is there extra experience you need to gain in order to accomplish various tasks?
* On the basis of your job description and the needs you see before you, what are your priorities in this job?
* What are your short-, medium- and longterm plans?
* Do your plans support, conflict with, or complement the stated plans of the organisation? (You will of course need to be familiar with the organisation's plans.)

Given the magnitude of the task, purposeful self-management – not to defend against but to accept, cope with and work with uncertainty and anxiety – is essential in those areas which are susceptible to good basic organisation.

APPLYING SELF-MANAGEMENT

Reliability

This is a good starting point. Just as one sometimes finds in a consultation or counselling situation that turning up and being there and being utterly reliable may be of the most crucial introductory value (and even be the most substantial source of or trigger for growth and movement), so it is in a residential setting.

Ten minutes reliable, protected and concentrated time with a child can be immensely more valuable than a whole day of snatched, on-the-run encounters. Making an arrangement to call on an older person in her room at 6 p.m., and keeping the appointment, is so much more productive than her trying to find you or contact you for days on end or waiting in because you said you would 'pop in' when you had time.

Reliability such as this is in itself a tool of productive work and, far from reducing spontaneous interaction, it actually promotes it. There is nothing worse for the people who need your time than never knowing when and if they are going to get it. They ultimately have to demand it.

So-called anti-social, attention seeking or inappropriate behaviour from children and adults alike is often a very clear response to unreliable workers or an unresponsive organisation. Whether it in turn elicits a positive and helpful response depends more on who you are than what you do. Angry ratepayers emptying their uncollected garbage over the Town Hall steps very often get an appropriate response and some favourable publicity, whereas the homeless person or resident of an institution tipping a few sticks of furniture and possessions into the street is unlikely to be understood by the very people she is trying to reach or influence.

The same goes for staff. If as a manager, at whatever level, you are supporting and supervising colleagues, be there with them when you say you are going to be. Give them reliable time: they may otherwise become desperate for help and demand it in a way which is damaging to them and to residents.

Reliability obviously extends into areas of behaviour other than good timekeeping: be realistic about what you can and cannot do. Don't put down three meetings in your diary, all of which you have said you will go to, and then go to none because you get stuck with someone who is enraged by your elusiveness and finds your ambivalence and lack of commitment to any one of the meetings a perfect time for them in which to collar you.

What are the implications of being habitually unreliable in one or more areas? It could even lead to having to give up the job and do something else, then perhaps realising that reliability is necessary, indeed vital, to most jobs which involve human contact (which most do!), and which put one group of people in the position of depending on others to get things done.

How can a lack of reliability be identified and corrected?

Example 2.1   Being unreliable

One of my first acknowledgements (and later understanding) of my own lack of reliability came when I was constantly forgetting dentists' and doctors' appointments for children.

I was working very hard, I thought, at all levels of consistency for these children, whose ages ranged from eight to sixteen. For instance, bedtimes included a story, quiet time with staff and a consistently firm but nurturing resistance to disruptive behaviour (see Chapter 3, Bedtime). Activities were planned with the children, and I was committed to being there with them to take part – for example, pottery on a Wednesday evening or cricket or gardening at other times. I had understood how essential the experience of adult commitment was to children who had been perpetually let down, promised, threatened and bribed, and who had learned from their own direct experience that people were to be manipulated and tricked rather than trusted.

However, my failure to be reliable about the children's health appointments was a significant gap in this consistency and commitment. It seemed that no matter how hard I tried, I kept forgetting.

The system of communication in this residential establishment was not the best, and my time was very short, but I knew enough of myself and of the potential for unconscious motivation to look further than the more superficial explanations. By working hard on myself, I eventually achieved an improvement in this troubling area of self-management.

The following questions are the ones I would ask myself now, though some of them I did ask at the time.

Self-analysis/awareness

* Is this a token area of disorder? Am I reserving some area which I consider 'free' in this increasingly orderly and reliable regime which I am trying to establish?
* Is this resistance much more to do with my longstanding tendency to resist regulation and control in my own life? Is this partly what attracts me to and repels me from the work?
* Am I trying to provide a reliable environment and stable relationships for the children and yet I collude with and approve of their delinquent and anarchic resistance to it?
* I need self-regulation as much as they do, and yet I find my own way of resisting the very thing I am trying to establish. Who then am I trying to establish it for – them or me?
* How good am I at fixing up and attending my own doctor's and dentist's appointments? (At the time I realised that I had avoided the dentist for three years and was not registered with a doctor.)
* Am I able to speak with someone about the difficulty I am having with these appointments for the children? Am I receiving supervision?

* How are such lapses in reliability regarded in this establishment? Is it a place where the *meaning* of behaviour is considered and explored?

* Am I relegating such appointments and the need for attention to detail to a despised administrative, boring, routine area of work which I think I am 'above' in some way, or, to put it differently, is not deep enough or creative enough for me?

* Or is this simply a boring part of the job I would prefer someone else to do, like the cleaning or tidying up?

* Am I somewhere harbouring the thought, feeling or prejudice that this is not the work for the third in charge, the *man* in charge of the boys' house? Is it work better suited to one of the more junior women on the staff? (I am sure I could not have asked myself this question at the time. It implies the exact opposite of what I would have wanted to believe of myself; so was I 'acting it out' instead of engaging with part of myself I had repressed? I would then, and even now, be angry to be confronted by such an interpretation of my behaviour.)

It would be by considering some of these questions, preferably in supportive supervision (but in fact for me at that time through a self-examining process) that a worker can acknowledge, understand and then *manage* and change such responses to common work problems.

The task of managing *yourself* is at the heart of all social services work, in particular residential work. Knowing and analysing yourself, using supervision, searching for meaning and motivation are essential (as I hope I have shown in my example of the dentists' and doctors' appointments) but what I have not yet shown is that at the same time, in conjunction and in parallel with this effort to understand, we must do something, we have to change our behaviour. Self-examination and increasing self-awareness may sometimes be sufficient to bring about change, but social work's reputation and image of agonised introspection is partly earned by a predisposition to inactivity and indecision. Effective management comes from a predisposition to informed, thoughtful, sensitive, feeling and aware *action*.

So one of the results of my failure over the children's appointments, after being reprimanded by the head of the establishment and following my own exploration of the meaning of this failure, was for me to get my own diary and start organising each day's work for myself. I have never been without a diary since (see below, Example 2.3, p. 37).

This first step in management, the understanding and management of oneself, is never a completed comprehension, but a continuing struggle to achieve a working competence. Only when a manager has gained an initial hold on this most personal changing and complex management task can she or he begin to consider wider management issues.

The five stories I tell in Chapter 1 illustrate the continuing struggle I had to manage myself amidst complicated and tangled organisational events and issues. Within those disorderly webs there were all the other actors, the outside managers, the users and my colleagues, also struggling with just as intense and complex self-management problems. This was true for Bertram, Lorna, for the assistant director, for Martin.

Tips for reliability

* Be there – on time.
* Make appointments and keep them.
* Use short dependable encounters rather than chance meetings or 'popping in'.
* Attention-seeking behaviour denotes a failure to give attention and requires a planned attentive response.
* Do what you say you are going to do; don't promise more than you can manage.

Reliability becomes a habit which quite soon becomes part of your working tool-kit – familiar, well used and exceptionally effective. The understanding and managing process, of connecting inner responses with practical applications, works. In the same way we use our principles and beliefs to guide our everyday work.

THE WORKING USE OF PRINCIPLE

While cultivating your reliability try not to get entrenched in your responses. This means not having mechanical and prejudged responses, and requires a real working familiarity with and commitment to principles. At every level in residential care, workers are taking decisions, influencing people and situations. Even deciding not to take a decision can be quite as important as taking one (and yet, of course, *is* still taking one!).

This familiarity with principles does not require learning them in rote fashion, but internalising them and making them part of your set of vital inner resources. Talk about them with users and colleagues; allow them to become common currency; test your and each others' disagreements until you know what you believe and what for you are top priorities. Then, when you are confronted with problematic situations, very often your actions and words will be almost automatic; you will know when something is OK or not. Although there will always be difficult decisions to make, your certainty and speed of response in most circumstances will increase.

Let us assume that some of your common underlying principles are to work for self-determination, increasing users' responsibility, anti-racism and anti-sexism, non-violence, honesty, cooperation and team work, unconditional respect for and acceptance of the person, and encouraging habits not rules. Sometimes these principles will seem to conflict and be put in different orders of priority. How do you use your principles to guide your responses and decisions? For instance, how would you respond to a person suffering from dementia who threatens you or a colleague with violent, racist and sexist abuse? (A very common situation for many Black women workers.) And how do you as a manager think, respond and act when a member of your team or staff group has just suffered such an attack?

How does a manager respond when a worker has suffered racist and sexist abuse? Put yourself in the place of the manager. Here are some of the questions, thoughts and actions which occur to me and which I (as a White male manager) propose in this situation.

Managing with principle

* Hear and understand what the member of staff is saying. Know that, even if commonplace and frequent, racist and sexist abuse is vile and deeply hurtful.
* Relate this one incident to the atmosphere in the whole place. Think about the inequalities in staffing, inequalities in Black people's and women's power and presence in the staff group (in the organisation as a whole). What is the context of this racist and sexist abuse? (Among the words which were used in one attack were 'Black bitch'.) Is this resident expressing something which is around (painfully obvious to Black women workers) but of which (as a White male manager) I have failed to be aware? Or if aware, have failed to take action? So to what extent have I not been listening to accounts of previous incidents or been ignoring racism and sexism that has been obvious to other people?

* Are some staff standing back from this and other similar situations rather than involving themselves, backing up their colleagues, taking positive steps to confront racist and sexist attitudes and language?
* Are staff given the time and encouragement to take their own action to seek mutual support and solidarity, e.g. Black workers' support groups?
* Consider to what extent this home could be seen as a service only for White users but with Black staff doing the work? Think about admissions policies and connections with the local community.
* Spend time with this member of staff and discuss related issues (above) with her. Make it clear that I have now heard and that I do understand some of the implications.
* Make it clear that I will take some *action*. I will personally make my position known and I will discuss and plan with the whole staff group what action we are all going to take.
* After discussion with the member of staff who has been abused, I will speak to the resident and to his family about this incident.
* We will record each similar incident and we will aim to reduce them by responding swiftly and unequivocally to individual abusers (those who persist and can be held responsible for their words and actions will be asked to leave or even be prosecuted), and changing the culture and atmosphere of the home so that it is clear that all staff and all residents will be treated with respect. We will review our progress in six months time and we will be in a position to measure our success.
* All staff will be responsible for making these changes and in doing so we will make the place better for all residents. I, as manager, will take the lead in this.
* We will consider the wellbeing of the resident concerned. What is disturbing him? What is his history? What is influencing this behaviour and what triggers it off? We may be able to do some important individual work with him which will enable him to be happier and more at ease with himself. Our attention to him and our concern for him will neither negate nor explain away any of the considerations or proposals above.
* *What additional or different ways of engaging with this problem would you yourself propose?*

It is in a knowledge of yourself, your principles, your experience, combined with a knowledge of the environment in which you are working and the people you are working with, which will tell you if a robust, unaccepting and even punitive response will be right (very rarely!). Or will the aggressor – young, middle-aged or old – learn more and be helped to change with an expression of love and respect for what *is* good in him, combined with clear intolerance of the words, actions and meanings of the attack, but unambiguous and practical support for the worker. It is always worth considering that individual incidents are nearly always symptomatic of a wider malaise which exists within the whole establishment.

ORGANISING YOURSELF

My long experience of working in local government bureaucracies has taught me that self-organisation is vital and yet rare. Bureaucratic regulations and routinisations have created organisations which discourage workers from taking responsibility for their own management tasks. There are managers, some at quite senior levels, who have succumbed to having their work organised for them, and have relinquished their personal responsibility for the way they do their own jobs. The larger the managerial span, the more likely hard-pressed managers will plead a lack of control of their time and an absence of discretion to choose courses of action and to make effective decisions.

An examination of their methods of work will show that often some have forgotten or may never have grasped the basic tools and techniques of organising themselves.

The hypothetical scenario given in Example 2.2 describes what might be found by an observer of a residential management group which works for a social services department or large voluntary organisation. It presents a rather depressing picture but some aspects of it you may recognise, or have had experience of.

Example 2.2   A residential management group

A small group of people work in the central management and administrative section of a social services department or large voluntary organisation; they are the residential homes section. They may variously be called the group managers, the adult or children's homes officers, the principal managers or assistants or the service managers, and their assistants be called administrative and clerical officers. Some of them will have been senior residential workers themselves; others may have a background in field social work or management and administrative work. The senior manager of this section

---

is likely to be a 'third tier' manager; above her or him will be an assistant director and the director of the department or voluntary organisation.

Half a day spent with this group is unlikely to give an observer much confidence in the practical, everyday management competence of the staff concerned.

Most of the managers and administrative officers have desks in an open-plan office but there are two smaller offices attached to the area. Some of the desks are occupied; people wander in and out; phones ring, sometimes answered, sometimes not; some people stand chatting. It is easy to gather the impression quite quickly that there is little purpose and direction to what is happening in this section.

If you asked where everyone was, what each person was doing now and what they were going to be doing tomorrow, you would be given very little firm information. They always have too much work to do; they can't do it all so it has all slid together into a huge and growing managerial bog in which they aimlessly and unhappily paddle around. Each time the phone rings or an envelope is opened the bog gets bigger, wider and deeper.

Crises are common and provide a much needed excuse to ignore or withdraw from the bog and to rush around reacting to events. It is clear to all, even to the management group itself, that these crises have their source in the bog, but that such reactive management is now the only way of prioritising work.

There is evidence of various resolutions to manage in a different way. A large board is intended to indicate the appointments and whereabouts of all the section's staff for the week; it has a few of last week's appointments showing on it. For three months the group has resolved to get together in a weekly staff meeting, but this was cancelled and postponed so often that they gave up trying. The same process undermined a system of supervision which was set up when a new principal manager started with the section. Forms were designed and circulated to record the work of each member of staff. Although their introduction was resisted strongly, they were used for a couple of months before falling into disuse. Staff realised that the information recorded on them was not being used in any constructive way, especially since they got no more supervision, and they saw that the principal manager had not used them to produce an overall picture and management plan for the section as promised. As usual, other things had intervened – as they always do – and the forms lie around uncompleted on people's desks.

This is the section and these are the managers who are looked to to provide the leadership, support and administrative back-up for the homes. But working from such a base they could not, of course, perform any of these functions to the benefit of the service being offered from the homes. Indeed, through their lack of self-discipline and their need for self-organisation and management, far from assisting the residential staff in their work, they fed off and weakened the homes' organisation. A group of managers who can't make appointments and keep them reliably, who don't have their own section meetings and supervision (and therefore don't respect and encourage the same vital engagements in the establishments), who simply 'turn up' and expect to be seen and to get deferential treatment, or are in contact only when something goes drastically wrong, is pursuing a parasitic and thoroughly unhelpful relationship. Their failure to organise themselves will be contagious and very soon the establishments to which they are employed to give a management service will start to operate in the same way as the central management section.

Grim though this picture is, it is possible to change a situation once its failings are recognised and acknowledged and steps taken to remedy them. As a manager it is not easy to interrupt and reverse the process described above – yet to do so is vital. Just as bad organisational habits are catching, so are good ones.

It is important to understand the performance of this section within the context of the wider organisation and its task, but that exploration is for later chapters (Chapters 5 and 6). In this chapter we will continue to concentrate on the techniques of individual self-management.

How does the manager in that section or in one of the homes managed by it go about the practical business of improving her or his self-organisation?

Example 2.3   Using a diary

For me the discovery and development of my use of a diary (about twenty-four years ago at the time of writing) broke through the self-management problem I was having with children's doctors' and dentists' appointments.

For all my working life since, I have used a very small diary which will fit in a shirt pocket and I can carry with me at all times. I can squeeze no more than four appointments in the space for each day, and in practice I rarely have that many. I write in only those meetings or engagements to which I am committed and, since I make a decision about what I am and am not going to do before I write it in my diary, I am virtually certain to do what *is* written in.

Although I often joke about my diary (and sometimes get teased for it), it symbolises several things for me. I think it is an advantage as a residential worker to be able to move quickly and easily from doing to planning and back again. I don't have to go to an office or to find a briefcase to make an appointment, or to check when I'm on duty at the weekend.

The large diary has become a managerial symbol and indeed a professional symbol (most social workers use one): but they tend to be divisive and exclusive, like files, clipboards, briefcases and now, increasingly, portable computers. And like the briefcase which contains little else but sandwiches and a newspaper, a big diary can sometimes be a bit of a front with large writing scrawled across large pages signifying very little but self-importance and the need for professional armour. You may have noticed how often such diaries get left behind and even occasionally lost altogether, whereas the disadvantages of mine are that it has fallen in the bath twice and I always have to buy shirts with breast pockets.

My own solution to my problem with managing myself in this respect is a man's solution. Most women and many men may not find this particular answer suitable for them. But if you are going to use a diary (and I recommend doing so), choose a tool that suits you and your purpose and don't be afraid to not conform.

Some diaries, and certainly Filofax-style organisers, do have space for the other vital parts of self-organisation, such as planning your day, and you may consider that the advantages of such built-in extras outweigh the disadvantages.

Making your own plans and managing your own time

The bigger the organisation and the more complex and demanding the task which is before you, the more vital it is to take charge of your own working time. Organisations have their own tidal systems, which of course you must observe and note and which will always have some effect on your own work, but to work successfully in such an environment you will have to be determined to have your own direction and priorities (taking full account of those changing tides) and you will sometimes have to go against the tide. (You will rapidly discover that the pull of this tide is far stronger beneath the surface than on it.)

You will need a plan for each day or shift. of course, this has to be constructed in conjunction and consultation with colleagues and their diaries, with users' needs, current events and issues, and the general diary in which all team members' appointments should be written, and also with an awareness of your own long-term aims. This 'to do' list should be made every day.

It is important to write it down, not simply to carry it around in your head, and to try to construct it at the same time every day and put on it only those things which you intend and expect to get done. Every day you should include action which advances your longterm aims. That may be a phone call or letter, convening a meeting or reading a particular article, but it is important to be aware of its place in and contribution to an overall plan to achieve a major change or result.

Try never to spend a day which is taken up solely with shortterm or reactive responses and activity – a few weeks of doing so will trap you in the bureaucratic bog from which only crises will lift you, before dropping you in it again!

Nor, ideally, should every day be crammed full with things to do. Time to think, ten minutes to stroll round the garden, time to have lunch or a cup of tea with residents, time to stop and chat, to relax on your own or with other people (lying on the floor or standing on your head!), time for less onerous work like putting up some posters or helping to move some furniture or giving a hand in the kitchen. Relaxed time is essential to a well planned day. I used to find that cycling between appointments was not only faster but much more relaxing than driving a car.

Managing your own work

*   Remember what you came into the job to do and ask yourself if you are using your time and energy most effectively. Consider this question in relation to both your longterm work and immediate work.
*   Know what *you* are going to do and how you are going to do it.
*   Have a longterm plan and move it along every day.
*   Make yourself a daily list which is achievable and includes your longterm goals. (Don't indulge in endless lists of things you might get round to sometime.)
*   When working in a team it is your job to communicate your plans and whereabouts to colleagues. When you have found a good method of doing this, stick to it and make it work.
*   Expect colleagues to know your business, and you to know theirs.
*   Be conspicuous about self-management – the more senior you are the more important it is.

* plan a time for dealing with phone calls and letters. Once you have opened a letter, deal with it straightaway.
* Reflect on your style of work – crisis driven/hooked or planned and self-managed?
* Support plans for organisation that are agreed and then give them a good run – don't expect things to work without effort and commitment. (But if you don't agree with them, don't say you do and then undermine them.)
* Resist form filling and all forms of extra bureaucracy.
* Use new technology but don't become addicted: that is not your job. Regard it as what it is – just a useful tool.

Chapter 3

Giving and receiving

As human beings, we are necessarily related and interdependent. Without each other we cannot survive, physically or emotionally. We depend on mutual support. All human life is communal to some extent and residential centres, when they are working well, are places where people can experience communal life at its best because they are given full opportunity – rare in the world outside – to organise themselves cooperatively with others.

In this chapter, I shall illustrate the day to day interactions of residential work, examining how relationships are built and how they can be used creatively. I shall explore the central idea that, as workers, we give of ourselves and encourage residents to do the same: we share and exchange.

Two aspects of the worker–resident relationship will be given special emphasis:

1 The crucial importance of the manner in which we, as workers, conduct ourselves in these complicated, day to day interactions. Have we acquired the strength to believe in the people we are working with? Are we reliable, committed and respectful in our dealings with them?
2 Close relationships such as we must seek to build are founded on very personal and intimate connections. They require us to bring to them our own lives and histories, our deepest feelings. Yet, we must establish useful boundaries to enable us to function as workers rather than merging with users. We have to keep our personal and work lives separate but we cannot disconnect them.

FANTASY/PHANTASY, THE UNCONSCIOUS, TRANSFERENCE AND COUNTER-TRANSFERENCE

In the preceding chapters I have been using my experience and limited knowledge of psychological and psychoanalytical theory to describe, explain and understand some of residential life and work. Such theory is, I believe, used quite commonly and yet, as someone without extensive theoretical education and training in this area, I am not at ease with propounding the theory – as *theory*. And yet I use it and, I hope, add to it all the time in my work. it is through this theory that I struggle to understand what is going on, for me and with other people.

In this book, and particularly in this chapter, I use it. I have to assume that you, the reader, are using your own accumulation of psychological and psychoanalytical theory to illuminate your understanding as you read.

In this chapter two psychoanalytical ideas are central: fantasy and transference. I do not feel qualified to write about this as 'phantasy' (which, in Britain, is the correct way of spelling the psychoanalytical concept) but I use the word in this sense – conscious and unconscious imagination, memory, images, hopes and a deep store and powerhouse of creativity which constitutes our inner lives and selves.

One important element of our capacity to fantasise in this way is transference. I use this idea to understand what is happening between me and another person when I find in her or him an echo or resonance of someone else who is or has been important to me. This is more than just reminding me of that other person: I find that I am entering into some aspect of my relationship (lost or hoped for or dreaded, i.e. fantasised) with the other person (often a parent or child). If I sense that a child is transferring to me his fantasy of a parent, part of my awareness of this can come from detecting my fantasy of being a parent to that child, and this idea is called counter-transference.

Such fantasies are neither good nor bad; like feelings, they exist. It is crucial for us as residential workers to become aware of them and to use them to inform and help our work.

BUILDING AND USING RELATIONSHIPS

This example is taken from my work in the 1980s as manager at Inglewood, a residential centre for older people in the London Borough of Lambeth.

Example 3.1   Dusty Miller: an emergency admission

By 1983 we had made some headway in solving the most immediate and urgent problems at Inglewood and had just begun to accept new residents.

At 4 o'clock one afternoon I received a phone call from our central management section asking if we would take in a 70–year-old man who had a broken leg and was living in a derelict flat. It was doubted that he could survive another night there. The other man who had shared the flat had broken Dusty's leg in a fight and had then set fire to the flat. The windows were broken, there was no heating or food and Dusty spent his time lying on a pile of dirty clothes on a mattress. He refused to live with his daughters, both of whom were most concerned about him and had been taking him food. He had discharged himself from hospital early after having his leg set in plaster and had returned to his flat. Some years before he had suffered a brain injury which appeared to have altered his character and behaviour and he had ceased to care for himself.

At this stage I was accompanying my colleagues on assessment visits in order to establish our new admissions practice. N o resident was accepted without an assessment by us, and we expected them to make a tentative decision based on as much information about Inglewood as we could give them. After our initial visit to them and usually a visit from them to us, we encouraged prospective residents to stay in the home for a couple of nights before they made a commitment to trying out the place in earnest. This complete process was not possible in the present situation and yet it was still important for us to assess Dusty, and he us. If we offered him a room, he had to decide whether to take it or not.

I happened to be the duty person that afternoon, taking charge of the late shift, and my immediate inclination was to say 'No' without any further discussion. Dusty sounded as if he was the sort of person who never fitted in to a residential home; the sort who would hate it and be resented himself. In no time at all there would be an outcry from staff and residents – and relatives. We already had a disproportionate number of rather difficult and socially unacceptable people and were not yet consistently successful at meeting their individual needs. Dusty would be one more. But he clearly needed the 'care and attention' which obliged the local authority to provide suitable accommodation (Section 21(1) of Part III of the National Assistance Act (1948), hence 'Part III Homes'). In spite of my doubts about our capacity to cope with Dusty, I thought that Inglewood might be the most likely of all the homes in the borough to accept and work with him. In any case, I also wanted to encourage the staff group to see our future role in much broader terms: actively opening our doors to a wider range of potential users.

I left a colleague in charge, acting as duty person in my absence, and cycled off to see Dusty.

He was indeed lying on a filthy pile of clothes on a mattress in a burnt-out flat; his plastered leg was stretched out in front of him and he was cold. I sat on the mattress and we talked. He wanted all the things we *could* provide even at that early stage of the home's development: food, warmth and a bed

– somewhere 'to kip' as he said. I attempted to outline the drawbacks of living in a residential home. I told him everything I could think of about the place, good and bad. I emphasised the lack of freedom which sharing a room and other facilities would entail. Dusty was not discouraged by these obstacles. As he saw it, he wanted very little and he would sort out any other problems as they arose.

I had to accept his decision. Having gone to see him and talked with him I could hardly turn around and say, 'Sorry, we can't offer you a place.' His need was evident and nothing I had seen or heard was substantially different from what I had been told on the phone.

The referrer hardly ever understands the full impact of requesting a place in residential care. Every new resident requires some of the time and attention which is being given to other residents. The arrival of every new resident has an impact on everyone else in the home. To the residential worker who receives the request it is a very complicated calculation and a major commitment. The state of the place, the existing resident group, the staff team, situations and resources which are in a constant state of flux, the near, middle- and longterm prospects of change and development – all these have to be considered when a place is requested. When you know that the prospective resident is going to be a particularly difficult person to work with, the risks and anxieties are even greater.

Even so, the worker who makes first contact must also see and hear the *person* – the individual in need – and try to respond despite the barriers and hostility which his or her wider preoccupations engender.

I liked Dusty's very direct statement of his needs and his practical dismissal of all the difficulties I was trying to present him with. He needed a room (shared or not didn't matter to him), a bed, warmth and food, and here was I prattling on about the dangers of institutionalisation.

I returned to Inglewood. I knew there were no single rooms available and we were actively reducing the sharing of rooms except when people chose to do so. I talked to a man who was on his own in a four-bedded room and who, I thought would prefer to have company. Much to my relief he agreed to share with Dusty. I got a bed ready and informed relevant staff and residents that Dusty was about to arrive. I needed to tell them about him but not to prejudice them against him. Everyone was very busy helping other residents to bed so I knew I would have to see Dusty in, to welcome and receive him. Having been to see him and assess him, I was also for that reason the best person to continue the job.

He was brought by one of his daughters in her car. They had stopped on the way to buy steak, mushrooms and tomatoes so that he would have a good meal, his favourite, that night. Although it was well after the time of the evening meal, I would of course have cooked him something when he arrived but this was an even better start. Buying the food for him was another way for his daughter to express her love and concern. While she settled him into his room I cooked his supper, which also established me in a caring and providing role.

I sat having a cup of tea with him and his daughter while he ate. Dusty didn't say much but it was a useful time for us to map out what he might expect from us – the staff at Inglewood – and from his two daughters. This was a symbolic as well as practical moment, as are most in these situations. I needed to explain to him and to his daughter that this was not what I usually did in my work and that someone else would be taking my place tomorrow. Dusty, in fact, got hold of this a little too firmly and always subsequently treated me as 'the boss' – not of him but of the place and everybody else. He expected me to sort out all his problems with a simple command, an expectation which sprang from his view of men's and women's roles. I was the only man on the staff with whom he had close contact, and I also happened to be the manager.

(It is worth noting that my attempts to convey that I, as a man, could cook and provide comfort and care for Dusty were quickly forgotten by him in the face of my 'managerial' role; however, it is also worth remembering that other staff undoubtedly noticed my direct caring role although on this occasion they made no comment. We men often get disproportionate credit for relatively small efforts to challenge sexual stereotypes! Yet real changes in men's perceptions and attitudes require much more than token forays into unfamiliar roles.)

I had left Dusty and his daughter to choose the clothes and possessions he was going to bring with him. These turned out to be a couple of bags of assorted clothes from the flat and an ancient black and white portable television which Dusty ran from an old car battery and which we set up in his room. With his permission, I washed some of the clothes for the next day but did not attempt to get him to change out of the clothes he arrived in, which were undoubtedly dirty. (It is usually important, even with adults, not to be hasty in parting a newly arrived resident from her or his clothes. Clothes are usually of great symbolic value – identity, ownership, personal connections – and the acceptance of the person with her or his clothes, or the stripping away of them, will carry a powerful message.)

The man with whom Dusty was sharing a room made no objections or requests about his own needs. This reflected his previous experience at Inglewood and his very low expectations that anyone would ever ask him about his preferences. He considered himself lucky not to be sharing the room with *three* other people and seemed to welcome Dusty's somewhat dubious company.

The next day I asked Chris to be Dusty's keyworker. She was one of the very best members of staff and consequently was too often asked to take on more and more responsibilities. I had detected Dusty's inclination to sit back and let people (particularly women) simply do things for him, with

> the implied threat that if they didn't he certainly wouldn't. Chris was
> someone who would not stand for this but at the same time had the capacity
> to truly respect and value Dusty, in spite of all his obnoxious habits!

In residential work we invariably build relationships through paying
practical attention to meeting basic physical and social needs. In telling
the story of how Dusty was welcomed into residential care, I show how
we got to know each other and I speculate on some of the thoughts and
feelings which were going on during that process. Dusty chose to make
his admission a relatively uncomplicated affair; nevertheless most of my
actions and attitudes were of profound significance to him. For residents
of any age and with a wide variety of needs and troubles, their first
acquaintance with the people and the place is of lasting consequence. (See
Chapter 7 which contains accounts from four ex-residents of what it is
like to arrive at a residential home.)

First contact with a new resident

Our first contact with a new resident is crucial; everything we then do and
say will be used to construct the relationship in which we are engaged
from that moment. Authenticity is essential, the display of the real you,
but also the real 'worker you', which on good days is the same thing!

A resident's life experience and your own are being brought to this
occasion and include early infant and childhood experiences and all
significant subsequent meetings, relationships and partings. (I emphasise
that this process is universal but in residential work it has a special
intensity and importance.)

At this first meeting we, as workers, are inevitably endowed with
meanings and memories from the resident's inner world (transference).
On meeting a ten-year-old boy for the first time, I possibly signify or
somehow represent to him a bad father or parent figure. This 'bad father'
is already in me (I can be a bad father whether, in reality, I am a father or
not). If I am working without some distance (a small part of me on the
outside looking in) and without a sharp awareness of my own inner world
(fantasy), I can respond only from that capacity within me to be a bad
father to this boy (counter-transference): 'This child really gets my goat;
he is annoying me.' I respond in a controlling, dominating and hostile
fashion. Our first exchange confirms to him that I am bad, a bad father,
and that is what fathers *are* like. My response to him and his reaction to
me confirm the other side of the equation: he is a bad boy requiring

a repetition of the dominating parent behaviour which I have just produced.

If this child is Black, there will be within him another, equally powerful layer of bad experience of the world I, as a White senior worker, represent. His first hostile and suspicious responses may not be simply to my bad father dominant behaviour but to the racist element he picks up in my behaviour, my demeanour, my words. I not only represent myself as an individual, but, particularly as a senior worker, I clearly represent something about the whole place he has come to live in. What can he expect from such a place? Certainly not an experience of a good relationship, like that which can be felt from a firm, kindly, protective, trusting and loving father.

(It will be clear that here I write only from my own particular experience. You will need to compare and explore your own different experience, for instance, as a Black senior worker, which will have very different implications and outcomes during *your* first contact with a new resident.)

Forewarned of the likelihood of such a situation between me and this child, having understood the roots of his hostility and resistance and acknowledged the possibility of my own, I will do my best to prevent these negative feelings from dominating the progress of our relationship. I cannot immediately influence the real experience and hostile fantasies which the boy brings with him, but I can influence my own behaviour. Knowing of my inner world (which will include the bad parent and the racism), I must try to use those parts of it which are going to give the boy a message about me which does not coincide with his immediate expectations based on his real and painful experience. I also know that somewhere there is likely to be good experience and that is what I wish to contact. He will have had some good experience of a father figure, perhaps his own father, or a relation, friend or a teacher. Or there may be somewhere in his background an idea of a good father suggested by religion, or a story, or a public figure who symbolises a father – or perhaps a combination of several of these – and it will be this experience which needs cherishing and strengthening.

My approach to him is as to the good and loved child. Aware of all my negative, inner-world fantasies about this boy, and holding them out of the way, I must contact and use my inner resources to be the good father. These are real resources (again it is irrelevant whether I am in reality a parent or not); this inner world of good fatherliness is built from real experiences as a baby, child and adult. As the boy senses the good father in me, he may begin to take back and modify his fantasy (which has its origins in experience) of the bad, and racist, White adult male with which he first approached our meeting. If so, he adds the relationship which we build together to his store of good experience, as I add it to mine.

Roles and relationships

I have described and analysed only a small part of this first contact. We could construct and follow a similar example with the child and the 'good mother'. As a man, there will be times when I am drawing on my inner world and experience of good mothering, and most often combining mothering and fathering as they are put together in parenting. In establishing my relationship with the boy (in my example above), it will be important to draw on my mothering capabilities so that I do not collude with the harsh fantasy of split men's and women's roles. Good parents, whether on their own or in a partnership, fulfil a whole range of mothering and fathering roles and relationships.

In my early meetings with Dusty, we were building our relationship on a variety of important roles. By my looking-after, taking-care behaviour I was representing parental roles. Dusty had assigned to me, contrary to my conscious message, his paternal boss role (he had once run his own haulage business). The obvious role of 'son' to a man who was almost exactly my own father's age must have had a strong though, at the time, unacknowledged presence for us both (transference and counter-transference).

In the whole of this discussion, I hope it is clear that at no point am I saying that the worker *is* a parent to the child, or a child to the older person, or, in a different situation, a sibling to the adult with disabilities. The worker remains a worker throughout, but we are using inner resources and knowledge – the most personal and tender and vulnerable areas of our inner selves – to do the work. This is why good residential work is frightening, threatening, rare, and why we need support, supervision and reliable, sensitive organisations in which to practise it (see Chapter 5, Supervision, p. 105).

BUILDING RELATIONSHIPS WITH CHILDREN

For some children in care, one of our objectives will be to try to provide experiences in relationships with staff which have been to some extent missed in early infancy or childhood. But how can we provide an eight-year-old child with the love, care and the sense of being held which a six-month-old baby normally experiences? Almost certainly not by giving them a bottle, dressing them in a nappy and rocking them to sleep in our arms. (One of the most remarkable ingredients of the 'care' given by Frank Beck in Leicestershire was so-called regression therapy which amounted to systematic sexual abuse.) But it is healthy for the child to seek these experiences in symbolic form or in some very close simulation. (There are many socially acceptable ways in which we, throughout life, re-create and re-enact infant sensations and experience.)

Observing children: what should we look out for?

How do we know what an eight-year-old needs from her relationships? We take care to find out about her, observe her behaviour and responses, and we notice our own.

We will see this child's needs in our daily interaction with her. How does she eat and drink? (Notice the way she carries a small pop bottle, which she repeatedly fills with water and sucks from.) What foods does she like, and in what form? How does she dress? What can she do for herself? What does she like to have done for her? What little rituals and routines seem important to her? What level of frustration can she tolerate? What is she like at bathtime and bedtime? What stories does she like? How does she sleep? What are her characteristic and habitual facial expressions? What physical attitudes does she strike? Does she relax physically and if so, when?

As residential workers going about the apparently ordinary but exceptionally delicate and complex tasks of providing basic care we can see all this, and much more, quite quickly. It is likely that if these events and activities *are* of significance then they may also be times of avoidance and disturbance. Eating, sleeping, washing, getting up, going to the lavatory, being close to anyone, playing, being still and quiet, relaxing, listening to a story may all be accompanied by great anxiety and upset.

Finding a meaning in 'difficult' behaviour: careful, close assessment

Our main problem, the major threat to our work with this child, will be what it was at the beginning – allowing our own fears and anxieties to dictate our responses and cut off the therapeutic communication we have been attempting to establish.

As social workers we need to experience and take notice of the effects of our responses at an unconscious level, to ask ourselves what we are feeling, to allow our unconscious responses to surface and reach awareness. What feelings does this child and her behaviour evoke in us? (Some of this work will have to be done in supervision; see Chapter 5.)

We also need to find out as much as we can about this child. Often we won't find the file very helpful unless we learn to read between the lines and we speak to the important people in her life. Be wary of simply accepting accounts of people who have observed and commented from afar. If we listen to the child herself, her family and those who are or have been close to her, we will gather the most important information.

With the child's help, we find out all we can about her family history: making a chart, recording dates and ages and discovering how old she was when each important event took place. Without a painstaking, shared assemblage of the life this child has led, we may be overlooking quite devastating events: the death of a grandmother, a move, a loss of job, mother's illness, the birth of a brother, a sudden illness, an accident. Is this child stuck with loss or bereavement? Has this child mourned and come to terms with some major loss, or does she need to continue or start the process now? We need to know.

And we need to pick up those allusions to this history which the child will produce either verbally or in some behavioural response to a situation. So much that doesn't make immediate sense to us, or can get dismissed as inconsequential childish fantasy (and there is no such thing!), will fall into place if we are looking to see how it might make sense to the child in the light of her history.

We should also, of course, take into account and take care with all aspects of the child's physical growth and development: height, weight, vision and hearing; the possible effects of particular childhood illnesses; her experience of childminders, nursery and school.

Too often we start from the point of attempting to mould the child to what we feel comfortable with, to a way of being which will make our job easier. This never works because we then tend to block off the behaviour which expresses the child's needs, and the needs cannot then be attended to. Knowing what some of the behaviour may be about and starting to work in precise ways which meet the child's needs actually makes the job much easier and more satisfying. We are working with the child and not against her.

Other age groups

These ideas and principles are directly applicable to teenagers and adults of all ages as well as to young children. For instance, individual and family history is so often found to be at the heart of the difficult, or anti-social or withdrawn behaviour of a very old person. Once we start listening to that person's story, allowing her the time and privacy in which to start telling it, possibly over several months, we are helping her to make changes, to bring to the surface long-buried wrongs and injustices, losses and forgotten achievements. I have worked directly with many old people living in residential care who have been traumatised by events in their early lives which they have never had the chance to speak of. It is not surprising that the intimate care required by some people represents a terrifying attack, recalling earlier physical, sexual or emotional abuse. And yet our response, as with children, has often been an attempt to coerce the resident into submitting to our care, forgetting that there are likely to be very good, but deeply buried, reasons for their panic and frantic resistance (behaviour which too often gets called and, even worse, recorded as 'aggressive').

Building and using relationships

* Start with realities. Attend to immediate needs.
* Build relationships by engaging through ordinary events.
* Notice your inner responses; by noticing them be in a position to use them to influence your outward responses in the way you intend.
* Think of the potential meanings and implications of each engagement for you and the resident.
* Be aware of differences – race, gender, age, class, culture, sexuality, disability. What do they mean to you? What might they mean to the resident?
* Be meticulous in your observation and your research of the resident's history. (But do your investigation *with* people, not behind their backs, and be very wary of information which has not been gathered in this way.)
* Consider the resident's experience and the dangers and threats you might represent, and vice versa. Tread carefully and considerately.
* Cultivate and cherish your own capacity for acceptance and respect.
* Think in terms of the whole person and the meaning of their behaviour as part of them; and when their behaviour is unacceptable to you, say so clearly but emphasise the acceptability of the person.
* Listen and talk; keep communicating.

* Avoid punishment and further deprivation for people who have little or nothing.
* Respond from the heart, reliably and authentically.
* Use key personal times for relationship building, such as bedtime, bathing, getting up, eating, etc.

Of the key personal times I have selected two – bedtime and bathing – to explore in further detail. The underlying principles and the recommendations for practice are, as usual in this book, applicable to the other times and adaptable to all groups of users.

BEDTIME

For many children who have had a disturbed and difficult upbringing, bedtime will be a time of high excitement, fear and avoidance. Staff, too, may get very tense in response to the children's contagious anxiety. As staff, we will wish most of all to get control of the situation and this may lead us to feel very angry and behave punitively. We may even send children to bed to punish them. Yet bedtime is when we can do some of our best work.

What I have in mind is a gradual winding down to a reliable, safe, comforting and very enjoyable period, a time when the child can talk if she wishes, listen to a story (carefully chosen), get some quiet personal time with her worker and go off to sleep with less fear and apprehension about the night and the next day. Imagine that this child, along with many others in the children's home, has never had such a bedtime. Going to bed may be associated with terrible experience: drunkenness and violence, being left alone, being very vulnerable, being sexually abused. For a few children and families this sort of continual abuse will be their only association with bedtime and bedrooms. Children with such memories or others for whom the prospect of wakefulness, nightmares and the vulnerability of going to sleep is terrifying will often want to stay up late, watch videos, tell and listen to ghost stories, and be over stimulated in some way; or failing that, they rush around, fight and shout.

Bedtime for children and young people living in residential homes should be carefully planned and should be a reliable, quiet and comforting experience. But how on earth do you achieve this in a prevailing atmosphere of chaos and over-excitement? (See Chapter 1, Lorna, p.11). The organisational issues are discussed in Chapter 5. Here I am concerned with what happens between the worker and the resident. By using an example (below) drawn from my own experience, I try to show how the daily practical necessities of the bedtime period can be so managed as to make a major contribution to the therapeutic element which is central to all residential work.

Example 3.2   Making bedtime a therapeutic time

When, in the late 1960s, I worked in a large reception centre where the children and young people slept in small dormitories of four, five and six beds, there was very little privacy or apparent opportunity to give individual attention. But by preparing residents' suppers (albeit with meagre resources) to meet their tastes, by carefully chosen stories and music and – most importantly – by making time to be with those who specially needed our attention, my two colleagues and I managed to transform bedtime. No longer a chaotic (and not always victorious) struggle to compel them to go to bed and stay there, it became instead a pleasant, relaxed – even an intimate – occasion. Because there were only two of us on duty for fifteen boys aged from eight to sixteen years, we had to plan our work meticulously and keep in constant touch with each other.

We always gave the boys plenty of time to get themselves away from whatever they were doing before their bedtime. One of us stayed downstairs making suppers and kept an eye on the rather stark and menacing communal bathroom (which was next to the kitchen) so that the children could wash or bath in relative safety and peace. As far as possible we prepared their suppers to their special order even though we had the most basic and limited ingredients. We encouraged them to talk and continue the winding down as they sat at the kitchen table; and we tried to sit with them for at least some of the time when they were eating.

Upstairs, we spoke quietly even when we felt like shouting, and created a comfortable, peaceful atmosphere. We had collected books and comics which were tidied and sorted daily. Music was played softly; once when we had a student who was an accomplished guitarist he sat on the landing playing. Each room was read a story or occasionally we told stories – and this appealed quite as much to the sixteen-year-olds as to the eight-year-old. Some boys liked to have a hot-water bottle, some a teddy bear or other cuddly toy.

We made sure everyone had got his clothes ready for the morning. Everyone who wished to be was tucked in and said goodnight to personally. We would spend five or ten minutes with individual boys sometimes, sitting on the floor by their beds, often talking about next day things which they were worrying about, a court appearance perhaps or any other kind of special event. When the lights were out, one of us then sat on the landing while the boys went to sleep. Sometimes we continued to play music quietly, sometimes not; but often a child would get up, possibly to go to the lavatory, or would call out softly and we would sit with them for a few minutes or get them a drink of water. We were prepared to sit there for an hour or more, giving individual attention, writing the diary or notes. The essential element was our reassuring, calming and, to some extent, controlling presence. The boys knew that bedtime would be peaceful, relaxing and safe for them. They could choose to have their own particular needs attended to in their own special ways at whatever level or levels of maturity they felt to be right for them.

In most children's homes bedtime is not like this, though a safe and comforting bedtime is a universal necessity: time to talk, time to wind down, time to feel the care and attention of the staff. Even after coming home at 3 a.m., having been asked to return by 11.30 p.m., this sort of attention is required or perhaps specially so in such circumstances. A teenager needs to come home to a safe and well ordered house where staff understand but do not condone. Imagine (or indeed remember) yourself as a teenager who has got drunk or has taken drugs, and is frightened but excited by the events of the evening. Then imagine the relief or reassurance of coming home to a worker who though being annoyed by being kept up or having had to ring the police to report you missing, is also worried and concerned about you and wants to make sure you're alright and settled in bed comfortably and safely, who scolds you but tucks you up with care and love, and says, 'We'll talk about it in the morning'. She says it not as a threat but as a clear acknowledgement that there is something to sort out and there will be a chance to do that.

Staff have to be exceptionally well adjusted and mature, well supported and self-confident to work with such demanding young people. It is very difficult to achieve this with one's own children, let alone a succession of other people's. No sooner have you got through a whole spate of staying out late from one small group of teenagers, but another group starts the same antics. There were many times that I have been too tired, angry and emotionally frail to welcome a teenager home at 3 a.m. in the way recommended above, but when I did achieve it I knew I was working well.

Bedtime checklist

* Think ahead. Plan.
* What are the evening's activities? What's on TV?
* What sort of day has each child had?
* Who is working tonight and who is the best person to see each child to bed?
* What happened last night and what, if any, is the pattern of the evening and bedtime at the moment?
* Make your plan with your colleagues and write it down.
* Discuss and agree an individual plan with each child that you are seeing to bed.
* Be aware of groups of children as well as individuals, and of their influence on each other.
* Be involved with them and know whereabouts, in and out of the building, they are.
* Don't suddenly announce it is bedtime, especially when they are in the middle of something important.
* Provide some break and transition between exciting and energetic activities and winding down to prepare for bed.
* Establish a pattern and routine with each child.
* Allow them to invent their own personal rituals, something which only they have, and by all means invent your own.
* Never use bedtime as a punishment or threat: you are trying to establish with them that their bedtime is something to look forward to and get a lot from.
* Use supper as a way of providing something special. Follow precise requests for 'an apple cut into eight' or 'bread toasted on one side, one half Marmite and one half peanut butter'! Cultivate your speciality, as an apple cutter, toast chef or cocoa maker.
* Wandering around with a packet of crisps and a can of drink isn't having supper in this sense. Insist that children *sit* at the table and don't simply hand out bags or packets of manufactured snacks.
* Use benign, individually tailored routines. Have an order for doing things: bath, supper, piggy-back upstairs, lavatory, clean teeth, clothes for morning, into bed, story, tucking up, kiss goodnight, light, door left exactly right.
* Always link with the next morning by making sure clothes are ready and saying who is sleeping in, and who is on duty the next day. Pick up any anxieties about the next day.

* Be careful that children who have suffered abuse do not abuse others.
* And finally, don't just go away and expect upset and anxious children to fend for themselves. Stay around; keep your eyes and ears open to prevent all your good work being undone in seconds!

What I have written above about caring for children and teenagers and particularly about bedtime is relevant to working with all other age groups. I am not suggesting you give everyone a piggy-back upstairs and read them a story, but remember the importance of bedtime for most people. Whether you are directly involved or not with helping them to bed, all workers have a responsibility for and part to play in making bedtime safe and restful for residents.

All the basic, ordinary activities – eating, drinking, excreting, keeping clean, getting up and going to bed, sleeping – are imbued with emotional significance, and it is on these that we should first focus our efforts.

PHYSICAL ASSISTANCE: BATHING

Helping an aged or disabled person to have a bath is often a time for confidences and disclosures, and the forming of close personal relationships. You cannot get much more intimate with someone with whom you are not already in an intimate personal relationship than helping them to bath. At best, this situation is initially merely embarrassing; at worst, it is terrifying and threatening for the person being assisted. Many older people's lives in residence are dominated and ruined by their fears of and resistance to help with bathing. Yet this excruciatingly intimate invasion can be transformed by a skilled and reassuring helper who communicates acceptance, respect, care and affection, thereby supporting the resident in talking about matters of deep emotional significance.

I can imagine the resident's feelings and thoughts going something like: 'If she can accept and respect, care for and cherish this old body of mine, the physical me, I think she may also be able to cope with what I have to say from inside it, when I tell her about what I have been through – things I've never told anyone before.'

For her part the care worker communicates in many ways: through her words, her tone of voice, the pace of her work, her touch, her distance, her physical strength, gentleness and support, the thoughtful preparations she makes, her concern for the resident's safety, dignity and privacy (making sure the door is locked), her deft manipulation of clothing and zips and buttons, the choices she offers, the bits she just goes ahead and does. As that highly skilful and sensitive work goes on, so the communication begins to flow – both ways.

Giving intimate care

* Prepare for what you are going to do. Have everything, towels, soap, creams, talcum, to hand. If you are changing soiled clothing, bring a bag or other closable container to put it in. Wear suitable (very thin disposable) gloves – a new pair for each occasion.
* Plan (with the person you are helping) in what order you are going to do things and where. If you often help this person you will have worked out a way that suits them, but if you are new to them take it slowly and methodically.
* At every stage involve the person you are helping. Think about how they can help you and how they can stay in control of what is happening.
* Involve another worker only if you and the resident cannot manage by yourselves.
* Learn how to use – and then do use – whatever equipment (hoists, etc.) is available, but remember you are still moving a person not an object.
* When moving or lifting someone, ask them to also help (nearly everyone can in some way) for this increases their involvement and control, and reduces the strain on you.
* Try not to lift with your back. Get as close as you can to the person you are lifting. Roll and swing rather than heave and pull.
* Most people will want to and like to help themselves – you are establishing a very important partnership. (Encouraging self-help will take time if the person has previously been treated like a sack of potatoes.)
* You will communicate a lot by your touch but talk at the same time. Keep asking, 'Is this alright?'; keep telling the person what you are going to do and what you are doing. This helps you too, because it means you do have to think about what you are doing and why you are doing it.
* Use the same words and phrases as they use. 'Down there' means genitals, and 'behind' means bottom, but people will use all sorts of different, more or less euphemistic or sometimes very crude words. Accept whatever they use.

> * Frequently you will have to tread a very fine line between taking
> over and leaving someone still dirty. The more you communicate
> acceptance and real care, and the more you are trusted with this
> extreme intimacy, the more likely it is that the person you are
> helping will allow you to help them and thus help you.

It should not surprise us that people of all ages choose these times of physical intimacy to make the most personal and emotional revelations. And while some dread being helped to bath, many very much look forward to the time and value it above all other aspects of their life in residence. It is obvious to me that people should have the choice of who is to help them in these circumstances, and that most would prefer only one helper rather than two. It is also clear that the private and intimate nature of the interaction and relationship is full of professional and personal dilemmas. The situation is threatening for the worker as well as for the resident. (I return to this theme and the defences which we construct to protect ourselves from the dangers of such relationships in Chapter 6, Resisting Hindering Organisation.)

SEXUALITY

The sexuality of residents and staff is a taboo subject in most residential centres. It – whatever it is – is forbidden! The message is 'No Sex on the Premises', and yet the place is humming with sex. Moreover, that same unrealistic message is conveyed in much that is written about residential work, where it is also a taboo subject, perhaps to be alluded to very briefly and in a rather lofty and detached fashion before being summarily dismissed. Yet, as all experience shows, for residents and staff alike sexuality is possibly the biggest area of risk involved in residential care.

I have been discussing and describing the building and using of relationships between staff and residents as the process which underlies all the work we do, and yet relationship in everyday parlance usually means a sexual relationship. If we deny the sexual and sensual nature of the bathing which I have described, we and the residents are in much more danger than if we acknowledge it, accept it, and perhaps occasionally, after great consideration and with critical support, allow it to become some sort of actively expressed sexuality. I know this statement may come as quite a shock to some readers but our current and common practice is to deny rather than acknowledge. I argue that this denial is likely to lead to illicit, criminal and terribly damaging consequences. There are occasions when sexual relationships between residents and staff are good and equal, but we will not be able to recognise those or to support the people involved (in an already difficult situation) if we drive sexuality underground.

First, however, I want to make it clear that no sexual relationship between children and young people in care and social care workers can ever be defensible. We have no right as adults, in powerful roles, in positions of extreme trust, to collude with, encourage or in any way initiate sexual relations with young people in our care. When we feel there is a sexual message from children, as there inevitably will be, we are ethically and professionally obliged to discuss our observations, to understand our own responses, to share our concerns so that the young person's care and development can be considered and enhanced, and to seek guidance and support on what action to take. We would most typically get this help in supervision and in discussion with our immediate work team. In addition, our concerns should be recorded carefully along with the plan the team makes to assist the child. Clearly, if sex and sexuality are denied and covered up we will not be able to use these avenues of understanding, support and guidance because we won't be able to talk about sex in the first place.

The same principle applies in all other areas of residential care: that we as workers do not ever abuse our position of authority, of physical strength or fitness, or of emotional or mental power. However, to deny all possibility of active sexuality between people who are free to choose their adult relationships is to demean residents and to deny their rights and self-determination. And to avoid or suppress discussion and learning about sex is particularly harmful for children and young people who should be able to look to us for information, advice and the opportunity to explore their interest, fears and fantasies in a safe situation. As residential workers we need to know about sexuality, particularly our own, and about HIV, contraception and the emotional and physical aspects of sexual relationships. I believe it is desirable in most residential settings (especially those catering for children and young people) to have a breadth and diversity of sexuality amongst the staff group, reflecting something of ordinary society: homosexual, bisexual and heterosexual people; different ages and family stages; single and attached people; very knowledgeable (and open minded) grandparents and other (perhaps younger) people with little or no substantial sexual experience (and who do not pretend otherwise).

The prevailing atmosphere encourages us to reject sexuality, to conform, to see diversity as deviant, and to keep our fingers crossed, hoping that neither we nor any of our colleagues are accused of sexual abuse. We bury our heads in the sand and then we are helpless when workers and homes are blown apart by such allegations – with terrible results for residents of all ages, for staff and for the service.

My first example in this section tells the story of a relationship, a working relationship that became a personal and sexual one. This is a common situation. It is useful to bear in mind in what circumstances all of us meet people and get to know them. Residents in homes spend most of their time in the home and the staff spend a large proportion of their time at work – in the home. Many (perhaps most) relationships of people who work are formed at work.

Example 3.3   A relationship between a worker and a resident

Bill is a pleasant and intelligent person with a good sense of humour. He has severe physical disabilities and he needs help with almost all his care: eating, dressing, using the lavatory, washing and bathing. His movements are often uncoordinated and sudden. He has lived for some years in a large residential home where most of the staff like him but find him difficult to work with. Because it is hard for him to make his wishes understood, a lot of them just give up and do what they think is best. Bill, not surprisingly, gets frustrated and angry, especially when he is being ignored or patronised.

A new care assistant comes to work in the home and notices what is happening to Bill. She takes special care to listen to him and quite quickly and easily understands him; she reckons it is her job to do so. She gets on well with Bill and he with her. They talk and even though there is little time or privacy, Bill finds himself confiding in her, talking about his life, his ideas and himself. Jean reciprocates. They are roughly the same age and remember songs and events from when they were growing up.

When work is being shared out, Jean usually finds that she is asked to help Bill to get up or go to bed, or to shower him. She is happy to do this and Bill is relieved to have her frequent attention rather than that of some of the other staff. Later, he is delighted that it is Jean who looks after him because she is so nice and treats him as an equal. If Jean is away, Bill is unhappy, except when he gets her postcard or letter.

Other staff are pleased that Jean usually cares for Bill, but they are also worried and even a little bit jealous of this relationship which seems different from the way they relate with residents. There is something about this equal and close relationship which is unnerving in a place where most relationships are not like that at all. Residents also have noticed and don't like such easy closeness; it is both threatening and tantalising.

People talk. There are jokes and the managers begin to mutter about 'over-involvement'. Some of Jean's colleagues are apparently very accepting, even encouraging, but they never ask her what's going on or seem to want to discuss it seriously.

Jean and Bill are both feeling very unsure and isolated. At first, helping Bill with intimate personal care was no problem; Jean was competent and efficient and unembarrassed about touching Bill. But as Bill became fonder of and closer to Jean, and she to him, as mutual interest and respect grew, so did their mutual attraction. Now when Jean undressed him, showered him, washed him and dried him, these actions had an emotional content different from before, and inseparable from their increasingly loving and sexual relationship.

Carers, paid and unpaid, nurses and social workers frequently have to cope with the, usually involuntary, sexual attraction and arousal of those they are caring for, and often with their own unwelcome sexual response to an intimate situation. This is difficult for both parties but it is made more manageable by maintaining a clear emotional or professional boundary between the carer and cared-for person. All workers (and carers at home) need advice, support and supervision (someone to talk to) to maintain the boundary and continue the care. (I think those receiving the care also need such counselling support, and even more rarely receive it.) The same boundary is not there for couples, one of whom is caring for the other, although they will usually find ways of making a distinction for themselves between giving care and making love. If we think about the intricate blend of care and sexuality between any partners, the boundary is never fixed and never clear; it is constantly negotiable and pleasurably explorable. The simple request to 'wash my back' is rarely that straightforward; even if one partner does just wash the other's back, the act of doing so is imbued with a whole mixture of intimate personal and sexual communication.

So when Bill asks Jean to wash his back it is cruelly insensitive and unhelpful, and a dangerous denial to insist that she will just be doing a job she is paid for and all that happens between them is the sanitising of an area of skin! In our example, Jean and Bill are a couple in some senses and yet they will feel outlawed, isolated and underhand, and perhaps driven together in their segregation. A natural and unexploitative relationship is frowned on and feared in their establishment. Are we to say that Jean, who has got to know Bill so well through working with him in a highly professional manner, is not allowed to fall in love with him? Do we then force them apart in some way, by moving Jean to another job or dismissing her for unprofessional conduct? And Bill? Is he told that his relationship with Jean is bad? Does he get the message that he may fall in love with other disabled people only or with other residents only?

There is no clearcut answer to these questions and no readymade solution to Bill and Jean's problem. Situations such as these arise constantly. Kept secret, they remain illicit. Discovered, they could cause one or both of the partners to be removed from the establishment. Either way, they result in terrible humiliation and loss. Clearly, what is missing in the home in which Bill lives – and in most others – is the capacity to acknowledge and work with sexuality and personal relationships within residential care. In a home where relationships are valued as the most important aspect of residential living and working, staff (and residents) will be given support and supervision which starts with relationship work. Jean and Bill (like any couple) would still have to face up to the dilemmas and difficulties of their romance, but they would have help and support to do so rather than be faced with hostility, fear, jealousy and condemnation.

This example is sharper because it has an overtly sexual content. In the establishment, it is experienced and labelled as deviant. It threatens the defensive boundaries which the institution has erected to deny the anxieties which such relationships provoke in staff and in residents, and to defend itself against them. (See Chapter 6 for further discussion of institutional defences.)

We have a framework of law which makes some relationships illegal and it is never justifiable or ethical for us as workers to cross those boundaries even when the law is unjust and unequal, e.g. the age of consent for homosexual men. Some apparent moral dilemmas are initially quite easily resolved by considering what roles we are performing in relation to a resident. For instance, we do have a clear parental role with many children and young people; if we overstep the sexual boundary in any way we become like abusing parents, and we *are* abusing adults. We must be aware of that boundary; to work with children, especially children who have suffered sexual abuse, we must have internalised the boundary to the extent that the children are *never* in any danger of eliciting or being subjected to a sexual response from us. We will be able to maintain that firm and totally reliable boundary only by acknowledging and examining the content of child/adult relationships, and reaffirming our experience and professional stance.

The second example in this section demonstrates the disaster resulting from a failure to acknowledge and work with sexuality in a home for adolescents.

Example 3.4   A young man working with teenage girls

Jim is in his mid-twenties and working with young women between the ages of thirteen and seventeen. He is an attractive and fashionable person and gets on well with the girls. He is very open about his active heterosexuality, his girlfriends and lifestyle. He is teased a bit by some of his colleagues who make rather obvious references to his sexual relationships and why he might be coming on duty feeling very tired. There is a lot of lighthearted, rather crude banter. The staff pride themselves on being open and honest about sex; they feel this is a good atmosphere for the young women who are resident.

In some ways it is, but the staff group has not considered the full impact this attitude may have on a lot of the girls. Jim is flattered by the attention that he gets. He finds he can get the girls to cooperate when other staff can't. The girls say they will do things 'just for him' and ask for a kiss as a reward.

His colleagues appear to condone this behaviour although several are infuriated by it. One worker who tried to raise the issue in a staff meeting is told she is 'uptight' and the implication is that she is jealous. Staff affectionately tease a girl who has a 'crush' on Jim.

As you can predict, the situation is disastrous. It is dangerous and cruel for the girls and very risky for most of the staff, not least for Jim, about whom all sorts of stories begin to circulate.

When a social worker from outside is told one of these stories, there is an investigation and the home is temporarily closed. When it finally emerges that nothing actually 'happened', that there was no substance to the allegations, the damage has already been done.

Of course, a lot happened but it was in the girls' minds and emotions. What happened was harmful for most of them, devastating to some. Half of the staff left the work altogether.

In this supposedly open and honest atmosphere, the girls were being treated by the staff as if they understood and could manage the very confusing situation presented to them. Most of them had already suffered family life in which there were broken boundaries and very untrustworthy adults, some of whom had abused them sexually. Their varied experience of sex had not informed them or helped them to make choices, or to be in control of their bodies. And at the home they were presented with another set of adults who dealt in gossip and sexual jokes which they didn't understand and who encouraged them to use sex to manipulate other situations. And a young man who worked there, a person whose job it was to provide care and guidance, whom they liked and found attractive, apparently also used women as a recreation: a very damaging situation.

> It is important to note that Jim himself, and the staff team, were badly served in not having the management, supervision and guidance which would have helped them to avoid inflicting such damage.

Residential care works for residents when staff build caring relationships in which both sides give and receive, and the interaction is *personal*. If we intend to work through such relationships rather than by rules, procedures and regulations, it will be clear what a frightening and uncertain path we tread. The regulations set down for us will at best signpost some of the way, but more frequently they are No Entry signs telling us where not to go (Department of Health 1991, *The Utting Report*); they will not help us to do the walking. At every step we take a risk, with sexuality as with our attempts to control residents and to facilitate their self-control.

CONTROL

The greatest concern of childcare workers (and teachers and all involved with child upbringing and education) is control. The effects of recent scandals, reports and the resulting official guidelines to practice have been to confuse and incapacitate many childcare workers. Not only are they made even more apprehensive of the children and young people, but they are frightened to do or say almost anything for fear of contravening regulations and losing their jobs. Real care and control (linked with self-control) are not derived from rules and punishments. Yet workers are constantly asking for more punishments (usually called sanctions) and clearer guidelines on the use of physical force (usually called restraint) with which to control the children.

Physical force and violence

As with sexuality, there is a widespread professional denial that staff feel violent, or inflict violence – in subtle and not so subtle ways – upon residents. Scandals of institutional abuse are parcelled up by the enquiry process, enabling us to distance ourselves from the awful things which happened. In order to discuss control at all and to make any progress with it, I believe we have first to face up to the realities of everyday life in residential care, and in schools, households and families everywhere. I have been guilty of punishing children (and adults), depriving them of something, taking away their liberty in some temporary fashion, or even (and, thank God, only very occasionally) of hitting them or hurting them.

And I admit to the same treatment of my own children in my own home. I believe nearly every care worker (and parent) with substantial experience has punished the people she or he works with – mentally, emotionally or physically – and, much more frequently, has in some way wished to punish without doing so. (In making these admissions I am not asking to be 'forgiven' – I would ask that of the people I have hurt – nor trying to justify or vindicate my actions. I believe violence in any form in this context is wrong.)

I also know that I am capable of loving and caring control, and of occasionally achieving the very highest standards of practice with people of all ages and needs. There are occasions when the worst and best are to be found in a single episode. (I hope my stories in Chapter 1 of residential work demonstrate how I have sometimes mixed very good and very bad practice.)

I do not believe I am alone in sometimes feeling violent or hateful towards people I care for, respect and love. I know that circumstances make all the difference to whether I can hold on to, rein in and control my feelings (my self) or whether I simply cannot handle the situation I am in and I lash out, physically or verbally. (I gave an example of wrestling, somewhat unsuccessfully, with such feelings in Chapter 1, Arguing with Bertram, p. 13)

When I first came into residential work I arrogantly and ignorantly believed I had the personal authority to exert sufficient control in situations which required it. When I quickly and shockingly discovered that I did not have such authority, I sometimes resorted to violence, or minimum force, because I did not know what else to do. It is all very well using minimum force with someone who is considerably weaker than you are but it soon becomes maximum force when they are big and strong.

With babies and little children we quite casually and unthinkingly pick them up, or physically compel them to do something – sit in their buggy, have their nappy changed, put their clothes on. We may frequently make them stay in bed or in their bedroom; we don't give it much thought. By a long process of development, establishing our parental authority, the growing self-control and self-determination in the child, we reach a point at which we do not use any physical control at all. For many children in residential care this delicate and varied process of learning to take control themselves, of themselves, has been badly disrupted or rejected because of a deep disturbance or upset, or illness or loss. Residential workers (not in any case the children's parents) must somehow stand in for the missing controls. We can avoid this personal responsibility by imposing institutional rules and discipline but doing so leads inevitably to institutionalisation and inadequate, emotionally flawed self-control. If residential workers are to engage with residents and facilitate the growth of inner strength and maturity it will be a very personal and risky process. Residential workers will be exposed to feelings (their own and the children's) of fury, frustration, impotence and frequently intolerable anxiety about the dangers that beset a growing child or young person. (It is very difficult not to be angry with the small child who runs into the road – if you love them.)

There are times when you have to stop children hurting themselves or other people, from breaking something up (usually something which is important to them), or even from running away. You have tried everything you know – except physical violence – and you have not succeeded, but you still know that you have to prevent the harm they are going to do. Your commitment to the child concerned is expressed in your determination to stop him. You put your *self* – body and soul – between the child and what he is going to do. You may be hurt and so may the child but you are saying, 'I am going to stop you, however I have to do it.' But the use of physical force is a crisis measure, judged at the time to be the better of two evils.

The following is written to give a brief impression of a very complex and packed episode – a lot is left out.

Example 3.5   Using physical force to hold a child

We are in the child's bedroom. I am saying, 'I'm not going to let you destroy your family photographs' (knowing that she has every right – in law – to destroy her own irreplaceable possessions). And then I take them from her – by force. She shouts at me and attacks me to get them back. 'They're mine. I can do what I like with them.' She starts to smash things and tear her clothes. I intervene again and hold on to her as best I can, trying to stop her destruction. I struggle and am getting exhausted but I say, 'I'm going to keep hold of you till you calm down'. She is strong and raging. A colleague and two other children have come on the scene. They see that although she is screaming and shouting still and I am struggling to keep a hold on her, I am trying *not* to hurt her and I am not enjoying what is going on. I am repeating, breathlessly, that I'm not going to let go, and later, as I begin to relax my grip and with one hand to rub her back, I keep saying things like, 'It's OK. It's alright. It's over'. She cries and then she begins to talk. The two other children have gone as soon as they have satisfied themselves that what's happening *is* alright, but my colleague stays until the crisis is over. She doesn't interfere; she's just there – for us both, for the child and for me. She too leaves as the child begins to talk. 'I'll be down in the kitchen if either of you needs me,' she says.

If such care (and control) cannot occur for this child in this place at this time, from a person who has made a commitment to face such an ordeal with her, she will continue to seek it but may eventually give up. At some stage, ordinarily in their early years, most children demand similar care and need similar control which will be repeated, and reduced, as the child sufficiently internalises them.

With an older, larger and stronger child such physical control is not possible and the adult must find other ways of communicating the same commitment and determination, the same stoicism and dependability. We can give the message, 'I know I can't physically stop you, and I don't intend to try, but what you are doing is wrong and bad for you. I am going to do everything I *can* do to stop you – I care for you that much.' You are likely to express your commitment in a physical way – the way you stand, the ways you look and speak – but you are also communicating that you cannot, even in this crisis, take control of the young person's physical strength for them. We are then committed to the same struggle but without the physical control, and it will be quite as exhausting and upsetting and it will take much longer. It has to be personal and there is no guarantee of success apart from knowing that such commitment will always be positive. Our job in these circumstances is not to give up on people.

Our attempts to provide control must be kept under constant review. Holding a child or preventing her from harming herself or someone else should be a transient stage. We must be very careful that we do not get stuck at this stage and that the child does not become permanently dependent on *being controlled*. We must also take great care that control does not become the remit of male workers using superior physical strength to avoid and negate the necessity of personal commitment and struggle (Senior 1989 p.252).

Control through personal authority and relationships

Example 3.6   Women with authority

I recall two women with whom I have worked. Both were physically small. One was in her forties and one in her fifties when I knew them. The children and young people they worked with had love and respect for them. They had presence and authority. One would say to large and angry teenage girls or boys, 'I'll give you socks!' I have no idea what it meant, nor had anyone else, but she reserved it for the worst occasions when she was herself most concerned about the conduct of the adolescent in question. As far as I know, 'socks' were never 'given'. I suppose the phrase reflected her generation and class but most significantly it expressed her disapproval, her concern and her determination, in her special personal, idiosyncratic way.

Younger children she told to sit on the stairs. They had to sit on the bottom two stairs while she ostentatiously continued with her business, usually talking with someone else or doing something in the kitchen. The child sitting on the stairs wasn't shut away somewhere or isolated, far from it; he was very much part of everything else which was going on but he had to stay there until Mrs G told him he could go. Sometimes she would forget and the child called out to her, or saw her going off somewhere else and called after her, 'Mrs G, can I go now?' The 'punishment' was symbolic; it frequently stopped a child in his tracks. He was required to sit down for ten minutes and feel the full weight of Mrs G's disapproval. Nothing happened to him; there was no humiliation or deprivation involved. Her reaction when she had forgotten and the child had reminded her of his plight was an amused but loving, 'Oh, you poor thing'. The original incident was forgotten and finished – dealt with.

The other small woman with great authority was a teacher. She could silence a class of thirty, very rowdy fifteen-year-olds simply by appearing at the door. No other teacher on the staff could manage this class, renowned for their bad behaviour. Most teachers were frightened of them and spent much energy and ingenuity inventing ways of getting control *over* them, none of which worked. Raechel never had control *over* them; she required – she expected – them to control themselves. They loved her, and she them. She fought and won battles for them, individually and collectively. She took them to the 'best places' and expected them to do themselves and her credit; they invariably did so.

I learned a lot from both. I aspired to this way of working, but it took me a long time to begin to find in myself just a little of the same capacity for care and control.

I think these examples illustrate the quality of relationship required for control which will inevitably elude us if we resort to procedural stick-and-carrot techniques. For Mrs G and Raechel, the stick and carrot were essentially their disapproval and approval – no more.

If we closely observe the interaction between workers with this apparently natural authority and those with whom they are building control, we will see that they frequently ignore remarks and small instances of behaviour they may have forbidden. The person they are seeking control with still has the freedom to object, to resist. They may grumble and mutter; they make faces behind the worker's back; they argue the toss and are able to demonstrate that they are part of a negotiated deal. So it is counter-productive to push people too hard, to demand absolute and immediate compliance and to forget that it is *they* who will decide how to behave. It is important that people retain their dignity and autonomy, and the worker with real authority can tolerate and even tacitly encourage this show of self-determination. We should not be too worried, either, by being immediately disobeyed; this too can be an important statement of autonomy which may precede the change of direction we were hoping for.

Our authority will come from being true to ourselves, expressing concern and disapproval in a personal and authentic way. In order for our disapproval to mean something to another person, on its own and without a complicated and impersonal system of sanctions to back it up, we have to build relationships on mutual affection, respect, trust, acceptance and commitment.

THE REWARDS OF THE JOB: GIVING AND RECEIVING

At the beginning of building relationships with residents we are likely to be giving a lot more than we receive. It is our job to give at this stage. We will be professional givers; we are paid to do it. Most people come into residential work feeling that they have something to give. (We often say 'contribute' because it sounds more professional and detached.) But why else would we come into the work? We give our time, our energy, enthusiasm, our good experience and understanding; we give our capacity to accept and value people who have been rejected and undervalued. And if we do not have something to give in this way, we are not yet ready or able to be residential workers.

And what do we expect to take, in addition to our money? Our motivation to do the work is likely to stem in part from something in our own experience: a sense of not having cared sufficiently for someone, or of not being cared for; of something unfinished in our own close relationships. We are likely to come into residential work with some unconscious motivation to put something right.

The rewards of residential work

* What brought you into residential work?
* What do you think you may be looking for at an unconscious level?
* What are your ambitions about developing your work with residents?
* What do you get out of your day-to-day interactions?
* What makes you want to come back to work after a couple of days away?
* What progress are you looking for with particular residents?
* When do you feel undervalued?

If we work in a particularly challenging and stimulating environment, where we have excellent supervision and training, we will gain immeasurably in skills, experience and knowledge. If we are able to make the contribution we anticipated we are likely to gain satisfaction and appreciation. We may well gain greatly from residents we work with – their humour, experience and appreciation. Just knowing some residents or being part of the changes and developments they make can give enormous satisfaction, pride and pleasure. Working as part of a good team, gaining the respect and friendship of colleagues and residents – these are great rewards. Fifteen and twenty years later I am receiving further rewards from still being involved with and close to people I worked with as children and teenagers in the 1970s.

Residents give us a lot by accepting and using the contribution we wish to make, and one of our most important contributions will be enabling residents to give to others.

As a worker in residential care it is common to feel like a servant or skivvy, very undervalued. Working with a physically disabled client with severe learning difficulties may appear to an observer as totally unrewarding. And yet someone working well will notice changes and responses which are imperceptible to an outsider but of inestimable worth to the worker and client. There may be a movement of the eyes, an expression, a communication which has been consistently worked for; a contact is made or an initiative is taken whereby the resident gives a tremendous boost to the worker. During the weeks of hard effort when it has appeared to be all give, the worker will have been discussing her work in supervision and in meetings with the team she works with. She will have received advice, support, encouragement and reflective consultation. She will have had the opportunity to consider her feelings in the face of little apparent success. When she reports the change and progress to the team and her supervisor, they too will share her reward and satisfaction; it is what they have been working for together.

Chapter 4

Leading and influencing
Creating and using vision

VISION

Nearly everyone I have ever asked has a vision of what residential care
could be like. At selection interviews I am particularly interested to know
what a candidate's vision and ideals are and what personal commitment
she or he has to making them a reality. When we, as workers, are
discussing a potential resident's use of residential care, we need to know
what they are looking for, how this move is going to help changes they
want to make and how it is going to be truly and practically supportive to
them. They are being asked to look into the future, to map out where they
would like to be, tomorrow, in six weeks, months or years.

Example 4.1 A care worker's vision

'I believe old people get a raw deal. I wouldn't share a room with someone
I didn't know; in fact, I wouldn't share with anyone, so I don't believe they
should have to either. I think these places could be really good to live in.
They are free to do and think and say whatever they like, as long as it doesn't
upset other people's freedom to do what they like. I'll be old one day, and
I want a real choice to use residential care and enjoy being old.' A care
assistant at a selection interview, beginning to express her vision of the job
she has applied for.

With users of all ages it is often more difficult to draw out and encourage
the statement of a vision of what they would like life to be like for them
in residential care. They usually feel themselves to be in an even more
subordinate position than job applicants. So we must listen carefully, pick
up the requests being made and ask people to expand on them.

Example 4.2   A resident's vision

'Yes, I would like my own room. Can I bring my bed – and my television? Is there a toilet near? What happens about food? I don't really eat breakfast. I do like to make a cup of tea at about 10 p.m. I don't sleep very well. I do my own washing – the hand washing anyway. What about payment? I've only got my pension.' This is an 85–year-old woman discussing going into a residential home with staff who are visiting her in her own home. She is expressing all sorts of natural anxieties and she needs sensitive and honest responses. At the same time she is outlining a vision of a service which will meet her needs. This vision has much in common with that expressed by the care assistant above.

The manager too needs a vision. A practical and creative vision ought to be one of the prime indicators of suitability for the job. It is the manager's task to catch and to cherish the visions of workers and users, to add them to her own, and to lead in their joint implementation.

Unacknowledged and unused visions become stale and sour; they turn into grumbles, moans, dissatisfaction and sabotage. Indeed, some of the most powerful destructive forces are grafted onto a rootstock of positive ideas and ideals. However, it is still possible for a manager whose own vision and enthusiasm are strong, working with patience, trust and belief, to reawaken the original visions of staff who seem to have lost all hope.

MANAGEMENT AND LEADERSHIP: A REASSESSMENT

'Management' is a much misunderstood and abused word. It is generally accepted to be what one set of people do to another. The idea of self-management (Chapter 2) for individuals or groups is not a widespread or well understood concept. To varying degrees during the grand corporate management of the 1970s, and the harder and supposedly realistic entre-preneurial management of the 1980s and early 1990s, managers have tried to usurp the function of management.

This does, of course, sound contradictory – a manager's job, surely, is to manage? But the meaning of the word has become narrow and exclu-sive, and the activity of management, thus conceived, is unsuited to residential work. All work, all human activity, has an element of manage-ment in it.

Example 4.3 The domestic worker and the director

The woman who runs a household with three generations, with several dependents, and does a paid job, is likely to be a highly accomplished and experienced manager. Let us suppose that she is employed as a part-time domestic worker in an old people's home. Little or none of her management experience and expertise will be recognised by her employer. She will be regarded as a low-grade worker who simply carries out instructions. She will have to keep her vision, ideas and feelings about doing the job to herself; her managers will not usually appreciate her contribution beyond the adequate completion of her cleaning duties. They will judge her by the extent to which she does as she is told.

It is possible that her manager is a young man who has little idea of how her job is done, and not the first idea of organising such a complex mix of tasks, activities, buildings, equipment, money and people as this domestic worker does at home. (If he does have some idea it is likely to have come from his own mother!)

It is also possible that this young man takes a management course (say, a Diploma in Management Studies) and gains promotion to a higher managerial post. Perhaps he even ends up directing a large social services department.

Let us suppose his former subordinate, the domestic worker, moves into full-time paid work as a care assistant, and is contemplating further advancement into a first-line management job. (As her children have grown up, her other very full-time but unpaid work in the family home has reduced.) In about the same time that it took the young man to climb to the dizzy heights of director of social services, she has moved from a part-time menial job to a full-time, but weekly paid and still technically manual, job. Not once in this ten-year period has her management knowledge and experience been recognised, used or developed.

Although our new director of social services may have learned from her when he managed her, it is unlikely that he will be aware of having done so, and he certainly would not in any serious or public way attribute any of his management expertise to this woman's influence. Unfortunately, his performance as a very senior manager is unlikely to display an awareness or grasp of practical management abilities of the sort that the majority of basic-grade workers in his department have to use daily to, in the official terminology, 'deliver the service'; indeed, even his language will be management-speak – quite incomprehensible to most of 'his' staff.

Meanwhile, the care assistant going for promotion to a first-line management job may be unable to acknowledge or value her own very rich and useful experience. She may have learned that the domestic management with which she has had such a profound and thorough involvement is not regarded as the management required in organisations, directorates and departments.

She has spent her life making things happen, getting people to live and work together under the most severe constraints, and yet even she does not recognise this as essential experience and skill for management in a social services organisation. She and those who are interviewing her may concentrate more on what she *lacks* in formal education and training: her under-developed writing skills, her scant knowledge of office procedures and her apparent lack of what we blithely call 'management experience'.

In social services organisations the overall objectives must be to help users to achieve some measure of management of their lives, to increase their control, power and choice. And yet we so often see that the organisations themselves reduce their own workers' control, power and choice, and are therefore unlikely to meet their objectives with their clients.

An organisation which fails to recognise and develop the capacity of its workers to manage their work is unlikely to be much help to users who need to develop their own capacity for self-management.

Clearly, the transformation in organisation and management which such a change requires will take place throughout the organisation and particularly at the most senior levels. However, the very concept of self-management implies and demands that each and every worker, individually and collectively, begins to take more responsibility.

Imagine two residential homes: one where everyone feels some involvement and responsibility for its life and work, where different people lead at different times, where users and staff share decisions, where roles and tasks are never fixed for long, where discussion is open and constant; the other, where the manager says, 'I'm in charge; I'm responsible for all you do, all that happens; it's my show. If something goes wrong, it's me who's answerable.'

There is a great disparity between the two. In the latter, no-one grows up, or experiments with responsibility, or learns how to lead, or gets the chance to make a special contribution or use her or his ideas and vision. (There were strong elements of such paternalistic hierarchies in both the Frank Beck (Leicestershire) and 'Pin-down' (Staffordshire) scandals.) Such places are much easier to run and are condoned, colluded with and encouraged by their external organisations. Contrast with them the residential establishment which struggles with shared responsibility and a democratic involvement in management, which builds, reviews and adjusts its structures from within, which agrees its ways of living and

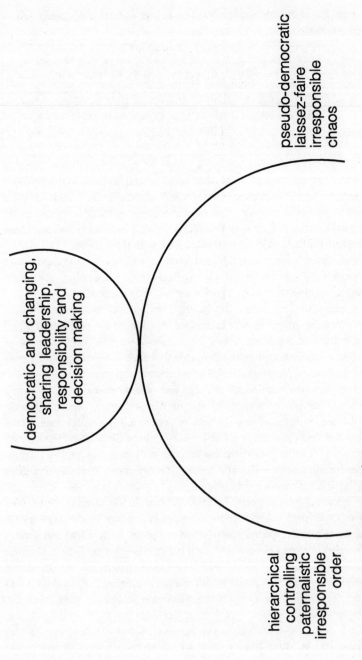

Figure 4.1 Three management styles

:ing together through experimentation and joint learning, which
ges as people change. This place is more akin to a good family than
₁ institution (see Chapter 5, Creating Helpful Organisation).

There are many places which use the strong paternal model (yes, even
sometimes when a woman is in charge) and many which make a half-
hearted attempt to follow a democratic and anti-institutional path.

The democratic style of management illustrated at the top of Figure 4.1
is most difficult to attain and then to maintain. Its maintenance requires
constant change and excursions in the direction of control and order on
one side, and of the *laissez-faire* approach on the other side. The art of
leadership is like a collective juggling act, keeping the democratic management of a residential establishment in a moving, flexible, sometimes
rapidly changing position, with an awareness that on either side is a very
quick descent into managerial domination or utter chaos (both of which,
though the result of very different managerial practice, are alike in their
disastrous effects for the users and most staff).

Taking the lead

My image of someone taking the lead is not of a designated leader in a
fixed role but of a person of inspiration and initiative expressing her or
himself to the benefit of a group. the ideas she expresses, the path he points
to, the insight revealed, are just for now. The group responds, perhaps tests
or resists the leadership, but a change and movement takes place. This
initiative is answered or followed by another from a different person. The
previous leader steps back, follows, and later comes forward to influence
again. If anyone becomes stuck in the leader role the progress and
creativity of the group will also become stuck.

The designated leader, for instance the head of a home or an officer in
charge, has also to lead in her own right as a member of the group, but her
most important task is to foster and stimulate the leadership of others. This
also is leadership – the promotion, encouragement and dissemination of
leadership behaviour, the creation of a culture of cooperative leading.

In such a leadership culture, the designated leader relishes the initiative
and assertiveness of others and measures her own achievements by the
extent to which the culture is drawing out and supporting leadership
behaviour from all parts of the staff and resident group.

SHARING RESPONSIBILITY

My discussion of management and leadership has a clear message about sharing responsibility – a concept more aired than understood, and very rarely practised. I start with a practical example.

Example 4.4   Buying food in a bureaucracy

A children's home within a hierarchical and bureaucratic social services organisation has a budget for food for the year. The responsibility for this budget lies with central management and most of the purchasing done within it (buying the food) will be performed by the administrative officers of that management. Food will be delivered in large boxes from vans and lorries which will call regularly, usually when the children and young people are at school or out. The main supplies of food will be locked away in stores and delivery notes will be signed at the home and returned to the central administrative offices. There may even be periodic checks on stores similar to a financial audit to make sure that the organisation's funds and property are being properly administered and guarded. (It is worth noting that central purchasing, with all its added administrative costs and lack of flexibility, is usually an extremely expensive way of buying food.) Any immediate, everyday necessities may be bought on petty cash, but their purchase will have to be justified in writing and backed by printed receipts; these will also be submitted weekly and checked annually by auditors.

In a residential home food and its associated activities are crucial to the care, practice and culture of the place (see Chapters 3 and 5). The procedures I have just described are appallingly bad practice, making it very difficult to use food in a therapeutic and positive way. Food comes out of a locked store; the process of obtaining and choosing it is completely separated from the people who prepare, cook and eat it. A vital element of their communal life is institutionally and mechanistically removed from their control (Rose 1990).

Let us now consider wholly different arrangements and the changed attitudes they generate.

Example 4.5   Sharing responsibility for food

We are still in a children's home, still with the same annual budget for food, but it is a place where residents and staff have full control together over what food they get (within their budget), how they prepare and cook it and how they eat it. They do not of course have a community meeting (see Chapter 5, Example 5.4, p.103) every time someone needs to go to the shops just to buy some milk or fruit, nor do they all do the shopping, cooking or washing up. However, the job of managing the catering is taken in turns by different workers, with help from colleagues and from the children and young people. Who takes on this very difficult job is decided either at the staff meeting or the community meeting, or both, and comments, suggestions and major decisions regarding food and everything to do with it are regular items of discussion both in formal meetings and informal gatherings. The food budget will be frequently examined and will be available to everyone.

Most of the children will be expected to take part in the shopping and cooking at some time. They will be used to budgeting on a large household scale; they will handle largish sums of money and account for how they spend it. The residents will be learning social and practical skills – catering, budgeting, decision making – which few of their friends and contemporaries are likely to learn in their smaller family households.

Although the food will be important to everyone, not all the staff and residents will be expected to take part in its selection and preparation. Some children won't be ready to shop or cook. For them, the eating will be too important to leave time and emotional energy for anything else. Staff are likely to move in and out of some of the domestic, household managing roles but the whole staff group will be wary of reproducing stereotypical 'women's' roles, particularly in connection with managing the food. The boys who live there, quite as much as the girls, will have the advantage of knowing about running a (very large) household and sharing responsibility for seeing that it is a good, comforting and nourishing environment.

I have used this example to show that sharing responsibility is not simply an ideal to be affirmed. It is a practical principle to be woven into the fabric of everyday life. People who share responsibility in their own homes know that it is a successful way of organising household business. Children do not grow up well in families which have very strict and unchanging roles and responsibilities; and it is well to remember that many of the children and younger adults who are living in residential homes come from families in which their own opportunities to take responsibility have been very restricted. (Or occasionally those responsibilities have been impossibly onerous. Responsibilities which should have been shared have trapped and crushed a child or teenager.)

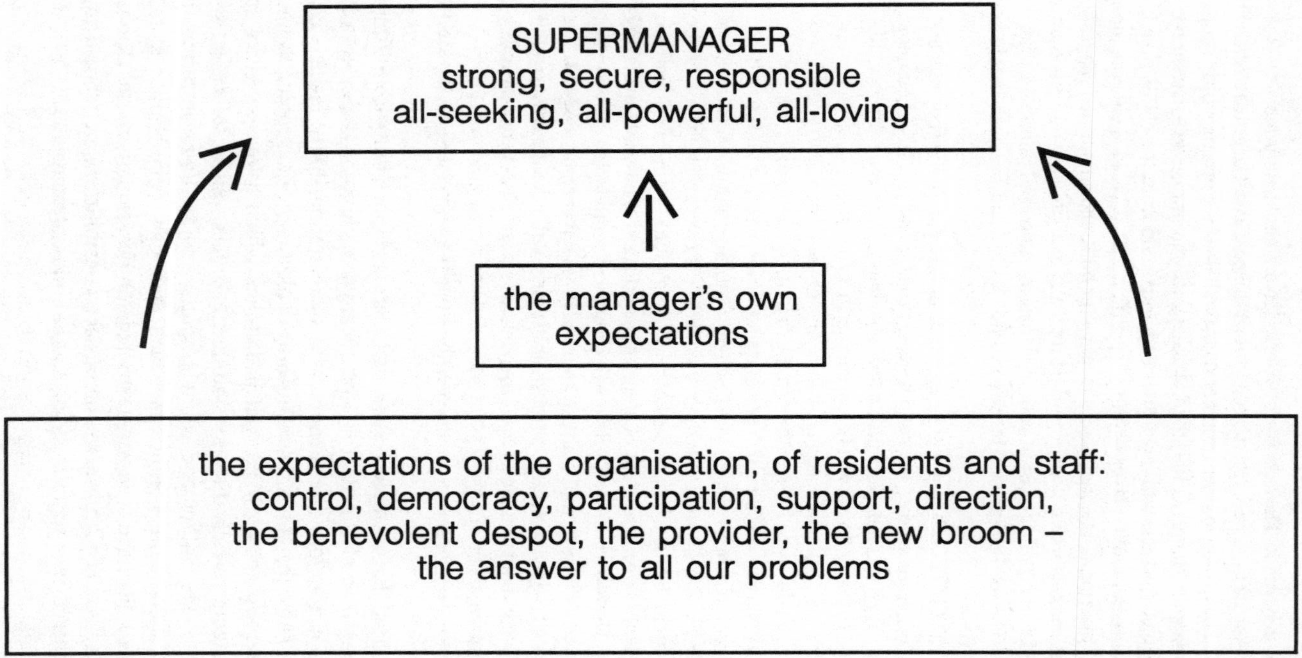

SUPERMANAGER
strong, secure, responsible
all-seeking, all-powerful, all-loving

the manager's own
expectations

the expectations of the organisation, of residents and staff:
control, democracy, participation, support, direction,
the benevolent despot, the provider, the new broom –
the answer to all our problems

Figure 4.2 Expectations of Supermanager

That is why it cannot be assumed that in a residential home the sharing of responsibility will be achieved by simply allowing a natural and ordinary set of relationships to emerge and evolve. Because of the limited experience of many residents, that is unlikely to happen. Shared responsibility has to be consciously and continuously worked at and the last thing the designated manager should do is to 'take over'. The management task will be the steady devolvement of responsibility and power.

BECOMING A SENIOR WORKER

The Supermanager fantasy

Such a flexible and constantly negotiable shared management as I have described above in relation to food sounds very difficult to achieve, especially if you have recently taken on new responsibilities and will have been told what is expected of you by senior managers in your organisation.

You will also have very high expectations of yourself. You have managed to convince the appointment panel that you could and would take on all the managerial responsibilities and tasks outlined in the job description. It is not easy to see how the performance of those duties, specified in hierarchical terms, can be reconciled with your own commitments to the principles of user participation and to nurturing a democratic staff process. As a newly appointed manager of a residential home, you are right in the middle of these conflicting expectations.

Let us suppose that you are seen by your managers and by the staff as some sort of new broom which can both sweep away and sort out all the problems of the establishment or team in the space of a few months. While knowing the reality, you too may cherish this illusion and use it to ease the anxiety and dread you have of taking on a new and frightening task. (I have been in this situation on more than one occasion.) There is a shared fantasy around of the exceptionally benevolent despot: the all-seeing, all-powerful, but all-loving Supermanager (Figure 4.2). (See Clark 1991, 'Supertrainer', p. 117).

Supermanager is not real. She or he is a fantasy – the manager we dream of being and being managed by. Supermanager is, however, always present – for the organisation, for us, for users, for workers, for the public. Supermanager is unfailingly patient and kind, yet utterly decisive and clear thinking. Supermanager is strong and gentle etc. etc.

Every manager is measured against Supermanager and found wanting. Some managers become Supermanager after they leave and the next person in the post has to contend with a fantasy that was in many people's minds a hard, living reality. Similarly 'Jokermanager', the worst and most evil manager, creates the fantasy of Supermanager, the new broom, coming to save the situation.

This may sound far-fetched, but the exaggerated emotional atmosphere of residential work and its amplified hopes and despairs put tremendous pressure on anyone who is designated to manage such a situation.

So how is the new manager to approach her job?

Some aspects of becoming a manager or team leader are different for someone coming in from the outside than for the internally promoted candidate. There are advantages and disadvantages to both situations.

For the manager starting afresh, Supermanager is a strong presence and an awareness of this fantasy both in oneself and in everyone else is useful. The following is a brief account in note form of the planning and first week of starting a new job as officer in charge, taken from my own contemporary notes of the process.

Example 4.6   The experience of becoming a manager appointed from outside

I had spent some months working with the personal and professional adjustments to do with moving from freelance training and consultancy work to very full-time employment by a local authority at a very large residential establishment.

I was giving up a life of comparative freedom and short-term engagements with organisations and people for a life of longterm commitment [I planned to stay five years], very complex and close working relationships and exposure to enormous demand from many people.

My family life would change. For the last three years I had been the partner with more responsibility for managing the household. My children were still quite young and I knew that this job would inevitably mean my spending much less time at home. And I knew from my previous experience in such a job the dangers of being drawn in to the extent that my family and personal relationships would suffer.

I knew sufficient about the state of the place, the conditions of life for residents and low staff morale to know that pressure would be on me from the first day. (Supermanager was already buzzing around.) Again from my

---

past experience, I knew that there was a lot that I could not yet know about the place until I had been there for a while.

On the day before I started I wrote in the front of an exercise book in which I recorded my notes:

2 days simply meeting people, reading, planning immediate goals.

Approx. 3 months – July, August, September – working on shifts, getting to know at first hand about the work. During that 3 months, complete an initial review of the whole place.

See everyone who works here individually for about an hour each.

That was my plan. It was deliberately simple. I was aware of the great advantages I had going into the place as a newcomer. I tried to make no assumptions. I wanted to experience the work and meet the people in the place, fresh and unencumbered by prejudice. I held on to the practice which I had developed as an outside consultant seeing things for the first time: retaining and recording my feelings and responses as instantaneously as possible, reflecting on them later; and not letting them shut out or distort subsequent information (see Chapter 7 and Appendix 3).

My notebook then shows what happened within the first week. My arrival provided a focus at which and through which to discharge anger, guilt, shame, blame, rivalry, jealousy, hatred, fear – a deluge of held-back feeling voiced by a staff of fifty-five or more and a resident population of up to 120. Outside there were hundreds more people with their powerful feelings.

The image of Supermanager returns. It was as if my arrival opened up a channel in a dam through which the pent-up water began to rush, faster and faster, until the dam itself was in danger of breaking up. Supermanager was expected to be able to open and close the channel, to deal with the flood and its consequences, to prevent casualties. I could not do that and fortunately did not regularly fantasise that I could.

From outside I received many phone calls – even on my first day – often about old events, long-running staff disciplinary matters (absenteeism, sickness, bad practice, even 'insubordination'!)

It was assumed that now I had arrived and the place was being managed it was time to start new staff who had been appointed months ago, and new residents who had been waiting to be admitted could now come in. This assumption displayed the strength of the Supermanager fantasy and also the unconscious destructive forces in the organisation. Saying 'No', refusing to collude with the fantasy, was very hard to do. Every instance involved an individual to whom promises had been (irresponsibly) made. I felt like, and was repeatedly made to feel like, the officer in charge of a crowded and sinking lifeboat who was repelling desperate, drowning people.

I said 'No' a lot, particularly to outsiders. While I noted carefully both what I was being told and the process, the way in which the outside organisation communicated with me in my first few days, I refused to become involved in many of these matters, insisting that other people would have to take responsibility for their own issues.

I very quickly recalled and rejuvenated old, well-learned skills of making myself regularly unavailable and yet being utterly reliable about the appointments I accepted or contacting people whenever I had promised to do so.

I insisted that outsiders made appointments (apparently not the usual practice when visiting residential homes in this authority) and I refused to be kept waiting if they were late (which they often were). I then asked them to make another appointment.

Nearly all this was done courteously and I was keenly aware of, and not unhappy about, the early reputation I was making for myself in the borough: the news got round that I had high expectations of reliability and promptness.

My focus during these early days, and for many weeks to come, was on the place and people in it. I did spend time with individuals. I learned everyone's name. I kept writing notes both as a record and as a way of talking with myself. I got close to some of the staff quite quickly; they were surprised but encouraged to find that I really meant that I would work alongside them and do everything that they did (see Chapter 1, Mrs Pollard pp. 4–6). I had to face the same practical moral dilemmas and unpleasant tasks which they faced. I had no immediate answers but I always tried to talk about what was happening and what I was feeling. I exposed my frailty. In the long run it did me nothing but good.

However, some of the deep upset and unhappiness that I was experiencing stayed with me. Several times, either at home, often in the middle of the night, or alone at work, I cried or was near to tears – angry, despairing, frightened – or revolted by the pain and degradation which I saw. I knew that they could not be Supermanaged away, but would have to be worked and struggled through. I also knew that we were up against huge and powerful institutional defences and constraints (see Chapter 6).

The experience recounted below is one of my own promotions. It happened a long time ago and I do not have contemporary notes of what the change of job felt like, but I can recall much of what was going on for me at the time.

Example 4.7 Promotion from within

One remark stands out quite strongly, related to me by a colleague. 'John's a good deputy but I just can't imagine him as head.' I found that hurtful at the time. I was in any case inclined to deny the difference between being deputy and head. I had just qualified as a residential childcare worker (gaining the Certificate in the Residential Care of Children and Young People – CRCCYP) and become a parent. I felt very grown-up and now, in such long retrospect, I think I was just starting a more mature adult stage which I had been practising for but had not achieved! I think this may have been what my colleague was picking up in her sharp observation.

I had been very fortunate to have been working with an officer-in-charge who was encouraging, supportive and utterly without suspicion or resentment. I was able to take a lot of responsibility, to lead in many areas of practice and philosophy and I never felt as if I was undermining his leadership nor that he begrudged my energy, ideas and keenness to experiment. He was a friend (and still is) with rare generosity and trust. These are qualities he passed on to me by being as he is. His generous support also recreated my own father's unconditional love and belief in me, which would not only help me to be a parent to my own children but also would now enable me to use aspects of parenting in my new role as head of a children's home.

The home itself was in the throes of massive changes. Several very significant staff had left or gone on qualifying courses; extensive building alterations were being carried out; being partly a short-stay home there were always residents coming and going. We were still working very hard on establishing our philosophy and practice of childcare and it felt to me as if I was left almost alone with this responsibility. Other important workers joined the staff shortly afterwards, including a new deputy who had also applied for the officer-in-charge job and brought with her experience, skill and a grasp of the basic childcare philosophy we were trying to put into practice.

As frequently happens in local authorities there was a long period between the previous manager's leaving, during which time I acted up, and my applying for and getting the post of superintendent, as it was then so absurdly and inappropriately termed (and still is in some local authorities – to their shame).

The delay in appointing me, my months of acting up, my reluctance to recognise the difference in role and our anti-hierarchical staff culture, meant that neither I nor my colleagues, nor even the children and young people, at any stage formally recognised and marked the appointment of a new head of home – me. And yet we did do this for other staff when they were promoted. Not doing so made it more difficult for me to accept and move into my new role (see Chapter 5, the use of ritual and celebration, p. 121).

At my interview for the job the principal officer referred to the home and its state of development after two years of initial change as my 'baby'. I noticed this at the time, partly because I was surprised to hear that she, my immediate manager, acknowledged the deep attachment and commitment I had to the home, and partly because it was a recognition of this parenting role in managing to which I had not yet given any thought. Although this principal officer had no residential work experience, she was a well trained and experienced psychiatric social worker who gave me very good regular supervision (see Chapter 5, Supervision, p. 105) over the next four years. Our supervision meetings were often stormy and difficult for me; I regularly tested her commitment, denied her knowledge and resisted her guidance. This is what she expected and accepted; this was part of her job and she continued to believe in me as a good head of home – a 'good enough' parent (Winnicott 1964) – in spite of my occasional rages, my mixture of infantile, adolescent and mature behaviour within our sessions.

Becoming a manager

* Beware of your Supermanager fantasy and look out for the ghosts of your previous Supermanager and her evil opposite Jokermanager.
* Make a plan for *yourself* for the first weeks or months.
* Plan your transition – leaving one job, starting another.
* Notice the changes to your personal life.
* Learn about the place by spending time with people – look, listen, feel, smell, etc. (see Appendix 3).
* Take notes, record; share your observations.
* Make your plan for the second stage (making changes) only when you have got to know the lie of the land.
* Be prepared for your arrival to unleash an overwhelming expression of unmet need. Don't get stampeded.
* Be aware of the way the organisation is operating.
* Don't be afraid to say 'No' – probably a lot to start with.
* Give clear messages about yourself and the way you work.
* Be personal and encourage others to do the same.
* Be vulnerable; put your trust in staff and residents, but protect yourself from the wider organisation.

Extra tips for the manager promoted from within
* Know that being head is different from being deputy.
* Relate your promotion to your life stages: reflect on the meaning for you at this time.
* Mark the change in some way.
* Acknowledge and use your own good experience of being managed and parented. Use the models you admire, without resorting to Supermanager.
* Try to create a partnership with your deputy or deputies.
* Demand and use supervision.

Parenting and managing

My example of being promoted from within describes a pattern and process of parenting which is essential to the good management of residential work of any kind. The parenting did not stop with my manager. The director of the department (Peter Westland) was also a person of knowledge and experience, a real social worker, who was creating and maintaining an organisation in which workers, establishments and teams could work imaginatively, progressively and riskily: they could develop. Again, at the time, there were many occasions when I mistrusted and needed to test this organisation. Of course, not all of it was good and not everyone in it was mature enough to understand and tolerate the necessity of such demanding behaviour by people who are doing immensely difficult and emotionally draining jobs. But there was a stability, resilience and liveliness in the whole organisation which encouraged and supported change. (See Chapter 5, Creating a Helping Organisation.)

At the time of writing, The British Association of Social Workers (BASW) has just proposed that nobody under the age of 28 should become a residential childcare worker (Watt 1992). I have some sympathy with this suggestion although when I was first appointed to the job of head of home I was well under that age and yet one of the oldest of the childcare staff. Virginia Bottomley's statement that children's homes would be better run if we employed 'streetwise grannies' (response to *The Pindown Report*, Staffordshire County Council, 1991) was met with some derision and yet I think there is great sense in engaging older staff, and my own experience of working with mature – even grandmotherly – people has been encouraging.

The idea of parenting in residential work is currently very unpopular and professionally unacceptable. Childcare workers in particular will vigorously deny their parental roles. 'We are not the children and young people's parents,' they say, with obvious factual accuracy, but with a vehemence which hints defence and denial. Who ever said that childcare workers *are* the residents' parents?

It is quite clear to me that what is at stake is the difficult negotiation and achievement of some good parent/child relationship. The processes which take place in any care setting – of dependency, interdependence, and independence – are embodied in child/parent interaction and are the essence of managing a good home.

Dependence, inter-dependence and independence

Throughout life we go through cycles of dependency. Most obviously and influentially, as babies we are dependent. The act of being born is our first experience of some independence, a physical separation from our mothers. However, our emotional and cognitive separation it seems occurs later. Again and again in our lives this separation and the experience of being dependent and independent continue. We move through dependent and independent stages and roles. Every parent has been a child; every parent has or has had a parent (in some sense). Most people experience illness or some disability during their lives which makes them dependent on other people for some of their day to day needs. And we become emotionally dependent. As we get older we are likely to become more dependent again in some way, but we may also adopt new roles which take back a parenting function. For instance, grandparents may feel very independent in some areas, may be becoming more dependent in others, and may at the same time return to a caring role for young grandchildren or even adult children. So these states of dependency are not usually static or one dimensional, and they are rarely one way in their direction of giving and receiving. If they become static or stuck, we are in trouble.

The grandparent wants to look after the grandchild. The grandchild needs to be looked after. The parent needs the grandparent to look after the grandchild. Yet, at the same time, the grandparent, the grandchild and the parent all want their independence.

In residential care there are similar dynamics. As staff we may be dependent upon the dependence of residents: their 'helplessness' suits us. Like any parent or adult child we are ambivalent about our children's or older parent's independence. The manager wants to be parent to the staff – to have them dependent on her – and yet also wishes them to be independent, to take the initiative, to take risks. At the same time the manager wishes *her* manager to look after *her*, to protect her, to be there for her and yet finds her manager's concern feels like interference or a lack of trust.

For the outside manager (Chapter 7), particularly if she too has managed a home, there is the temptation to take over. She may rationalise this by 'giving the manager a break' (from the children?) or by needing to intervene before the staff and residents are harmed by an inexpert head of home (youthful parent?).

The management of residential care not only has many parallels with family dynamics but is in many senses a setting for the acting out of family dynamics. Each resident, member of staff and manager brings her family experience into this setting and finds an arena already set up. Each person can watch, take part, experiment and improvise new scenes of family drama. For staff, an awareness of one's own dynamics and motivation is vital in helping residents to use this arena productively. staff group work and supervision (Chapter 5) are essential to gaining such awareness.

Chapter 5

Creating helpful organisation

IT'S NOT SO MUCH THE BUILDING AS THE WAY YOU USE IT

Most of the buildings which are used as residential care centres are in some ways unsuitable. They were built for another purpose; they are old and need modernising; or they are new but badly designed. I don't think any building of any sort ever exactly suits its use. The use of a building changes according to the needs of its inhabitants and it evolves over time.

Since the registration and inspection of homes has been compulsory much emphasis has been placed on the size of rooms, the number of toilets and a host of other measurements which are only superficially relevant to the care provided. Since the new 'arms-length' inspection teams have been established, some inspectors have begun to look much deeper than these superficial indicators and have been encouraged to do so by their local authorities and the Department of Health (see reports such as *Homes Are For Living In*, Department of Health 1989b). Of course the standard of physical provision is important – that is what the first part of this chapter is about – but as with all other aspects of residential care we need to be attuned to the meaning of what we see, not simply the outward appearance.

I believe that it is more than a coincidence that the two buildings of which I have been manager for lengthy periods were both opened in 1964. One, Frogmore (the children's home), originally two separate houses, was an early design of James Stirling, a controversial architect of international repute. The other, Inglewood (a very large old people's home), has an overall design common to several other similar homes built all over London in the early and mid-1960s. These homes were major investments by the old London County Council (LCC), opened and then handed over to the new London Borough Councils with the end of the LCC in 1965. They both were opened with pride and some fanfare. Amongst the impressive list of politicians, church people and well-known public figures at the opening of Inglewood were the Bishop of Southwark and Mary Wilson, wife of the incoming Prime Minister of the time.

However, both places maintained their pride and high profile for a relatively short time before lapsing into bad practice and crumbling, uncared-for fabric. I think part of the attraction of both for me (although I was not conscious of it either time) was the notion of a basically good place falling from grace but having the potential to regain its former idealism and position.

The majority of residential workers and managers in organisations which provide residential care complain that their jobs are made doubly difficult because of the buildings – the design, the maintenance, the leaky roofs, the institutional look. All these factors were put forward as reasons why the two homes I have described above could not function properly. In my own view, the building is rarely a reason for poor care but it is sometimes a symptom of poor care.

In both of these homes we had to struggle to improve the physical provision as we improved the standard of social work. They went together. We as staff had to start seeing and experiencing aspects of the building as 'good' or 'good enough', and making individual and collective statements of a new attitude.

If the building, furniture and decoration were so bad, what were we doing allowing residents to live in conditions which were spiritually, culturally and aesthetically impoverishing? What sort of respect did we have for ourselves working there?

Yes, some of the rooms were too small or some were cold and inhospitable, surely just as in any home, house or flat, and certainly as in some of those in which residents would have formerly lived. The point was what we, staff and residents, could do about it. That might involve demanding some major alteration, but usually we would have to find a way of making that room nice to be in.

Example 5.1 Involving everyone in changing the home

At Inglewood, when we started 'group living' on one of the four floors (without any of the structural alterations or replacement furniture which we eventually got by demanding them), the staff team who had been chosen for the task of setting up this new venture responded much as they would if they themselves were moving into a new home. They looked at the worst areas, in this case the lavatories, and decorated them. They brought in things from their own homes: ornaments, lights, bits of furniture. They begged, borrowed and... well, they acquired the equipment they needed. They badgered and persuaded. They involved residents' relatives. Everyone was involved with creating a home (one floor of a large building) out of almost nothing.

Relatives decorated bedrooms and also brought in furniture. There was a china cabinet in the sitting room to which some people entrusted their valued ornaments. Pictures went up. Everyone got involved with creating a home out of part of an institution.

Similarly at Frogmore, the children's home, when major alterations and refurbishment were being done we did not allow the local authority to provide everything. We spent months setting up home, making some furniture, repainting and adapting, choosing chairs and equipment and putting our mark on the place, all of us – residents and staff. (See Chapter 1, Martin and the garden, p. 16–17.)

The essence of what I am saying will be obvious from our own experience of our own households. Most of us express, live and anchor ourselves in various ways through and in our surroundings, our homes. The feel and ambience of our home is built up over time. A hotel cannot provide a home in this sense. We will have wasted irrelevant energy if we try to get the physical provision to the 'right' standard without making the connections between our controlling, influencing and designing our own environment and our own wellbeing – either as workers or residents.

Good quality and natural materials

Institutionalisation often deprives people of contact with the natural world. They are surrounded by artificial substances; they may rarely get out, feel the wind on their faces, touch plants or feel the ground beneath their feet. They may never smell food being cooked or see it being prepared. These are major deprivations which cut people off from the world. We must design ordinary life in the residential home to afford residents and staff contact with good things to touch, smell, eat, sit on, lie on and have around.

It is too easy to furnish a home with plastic, nylon, vinyl, stainless steel and polyester. A favourite chair, for people of all ages, is unlikely to be something which was injection moulded or is one of four dozen similar chairs in the home. It might be a new, wooden rocking chair with a comfortable cushion, or a small upright armchair with a footstool, or a large, springy, capacious armchair which you can curl up in, or an old-fashioned leather-covered armchair. (These are all real examples of chairs which I remember residents adopting.) A favourite chair is not necessarily in first-class condition; it may need reupholstering or recovering and the person 'whose chair it is', who has adopted it as her own (or it may really be her own) is reluctant to allow it to go for attention.

We should look for natural materials – wood, linen, cotton, wool – wherever possible and practicable. Colour and design are important too. Residents and staff may wish to establish a different ambience for each room. We will choose furniture which does not fall apart and is made in such a way that it can be mended if it is damaged or worn. This sort of furniture has usually been made (at least in part) by hand, by another human being.

An upset child is quite likely to damage something she or he values and knows is valued. If the episode is followed by the favourite chair being thrown away, the child being punished or fined, this is a depriving and repressive response. But if the child can reinstate the chair to its previous condition, possibly paying for the materials to do so and being helped to put things right again, this is a marvellously restorative and strengthening experience, and also gives the child the opportunity of acquiring very useful skills and attitudes for later life. That cannot be done with an injection-moulded chair which will attract a very different sort of damage in the first place – wanton and random destruction rather than precisely directed and significant damage. (See the chapter on 'Some aspects of damage and restitution' in Barbara Dockar-Drysdale 1974.)

Making connections

It is evident that the way furniture and decoration is chosen is important. Differences in class and culture and taste are real and very personal. There is an opportunity in most residential homes to mix and savour differences. Some people will want a text on the wall or a carpet in the bathroom; some will want plain wallpaper and others heavily patterned. Bright colours, gold and frills are to some people's taste and tradition, whereas others will opt for plain and muted colours. There should be room for individual choice and group decision making.

People's own rooms should be the way they want them, as long as their choice does not restrict or dictate anyone else's. In my description of Bertram's room (Chapter 1) it is clear that he had gone rather beyond the limit by stripping his room of the boxing which covered the pipework and discarding his mattress – we constantly remonstrated with him over these excesses – but it is also clear that he was making choices and was still in control of the way his room looked. It had to be restored to ordinary standards for the next person to occupy it, but this was not a hugely expensive job nor was it any different from the maintenance carried out between tenancies in other rented accommodation.

Reasonable prices and making decisions

Of course, cost is a major consideration when buying furniture or redecorating. It is anywhere for almost anyone. We have to work to a budget whether in our own homes or in residential care. In a residential home the budget has to provide for a good basic standard. No-one can be expected to move into a room which is in urgent need of decoration or in which the furniture is falling to pieces. But when we are choosing furniture or deciding to buy some new curtains for the sitting room, we need to know how much we have got to spend. Still, in far too many residential homes, these decisions are made by people altogether outside the home or by managers within the home. It is not good enough merely to consult residents – they are a part of the decision making. (See Chapter 4, pp. 75–80)

I recognise that decorations decided by a committee may result in a different colour on each wall and a carpet which clashes with the curtains; indeed, it may result in a style that is not to anyone's taste – no better than allowing the managers or administrators to decide. But making decisions of this sort is not always best done simply by counting votes in committees.

The residents may decide to delegate one of themselves or a member of staff, or both, to put forward a plan or alternative proposals to them. In any case, many of the decisions will be small incremental ones like, 'Shall we get the ceiling repainted this year?' or 'Shall we buy that clock or mirror?'

In short-term and respite-care places it is not easy to give residents the responsibility for taking such decisions but all the information should be made available to them if they wish to take part. They will be able to make choices and influence decisions too. Showing a particular preference for one room or making it clear that they do not like another will be useful starting points to ask them what suits them and why, and to ask them what they suggest can be done about their comments. This discussion should not be restricted to residents but can be widened to relatives and other carers, especially when residents may not be able to express clearly their likes and dislikes in such matters as decoration and furniture.

Physical appearance and provision is a very useful tool through which to involve relatives and carers in a practical and tangible way. It is a great relief to a son or daughter or parent to be able to take part in creating a good place for the person they have cared for. A caring relationship is very difficult to rebuild or maintain if there is no ordinary and concrete way of expressing care; merely visiting can be a sterile and embarrassing process.

Durability and the opportunity to care for things

It is important to convey a feeling and message of durability in the fabric of the home. A building which looks solid and dependable, furniture which has been built to last (not merely manufactured to resist vandalism), a carpet which is worn but not worn out – they all have important messages for residents. The way the furniture is looked after, the smell of polish, the maintaining, restoring and repairing of the fabric, never leaving something looking uncared for, a pride in the look of the place, wanting it to be clean, hospitable and comfortable when a visitor comes, welcoming the compliments, 'Oh, I do like this room': all these give a sense of permanence and self-respect.

Example 5.2   A significant sideboard

Children remember the large old sideboard which the domestic worker loved to polish, and one child took the same pleasure in polishing it herself. She looked at the way it was made, the brass hinges, the oak lined drawers, the carving on the door panels – somebody made this a long time ago and it's still here, and she now looks after it. When she revisits the home years after she's left the sideboard brings back vivid memories, symbolising a lot of the good experience she had when she lived at the home. Later in life, she buys good secondhand and old furniture; she takes great care of it, and her children grow up with it.

Pictures

The pictures on the walls are a powerful statement of cultural connections in the place. They can reflect, respond to and reach out to the mix of people who live in or have connections with the home.

First there should be photographs of the people and their activities; preferably not dog-eared pictures of the Christmas party two years ago sellotaped to flaking paintwork. Recent photographs mounted carefully on a board and older ones properly framed and displayed as we would important family pictures at home. You can tell a lot about the internal culture of the place from these photographs. Sometimes, unfortunately, they are staff centred, showing staff enjoying themselves with residents very much in the background if they are in the picture at all. Others may show residents at the centre of the activity but have staff standing around in literally superior positions, standing over residents (particularly if they are in wheelchairs) maybe smiling at them in a patronising fashion. Pictures which show residents and staff as people in their own right, equal and self-confident, are pictures worth seeing.

Example 5.3   Every picture tells a story

I recall two examples of how displays of photographs gave strong messages about the culture and internal politics of two establishments. In one there was a collection of pictures of staff with their names and positions written underneath. However, there were no pictures of any of the Black staff who comprised about a third of the workforce. It emerged very quickly to me, as a visitor, that there were many problems of racism here: overt racism from residents and the constant undermining of Black staff by managers. The pictures said it all, tacitly approving and supporting the discrimination and oppression.

In the other example, the pictures of the staff group were arranged in their hierarchy, as in a simple organisation chart: the manager at the top – a man; three assistant managers next – men; and ten other staff on the bottom row – all but two, women. When I drew attention to this, it was clear that the manager was unaware of the message which the pictures were giving and he responded by saying that he thought they had got the balance of men and women just about right although the women were in a slight majority.

I, too, fifteen years ago, have been in a position where the three most senior staff were White men, but at least we were aware of the drawbacks and worked to counter the short-term effects and make changes in the long term. I do not believe we would have proclaimed and, by implication, approved this inequality by illustrating it as if we were proud of it.

When we put pictures on the wall we are usually in some way strengthening and affirming something which they communicate or illustrate.

Pictures which have been made by the people who live and work in the home, nicely displayed, preferably framed, are a great source of pride and affirmation and are very likely to reflect the cultural mix of residents and staff.

Finally, the pictures which have been created elsewhere. When working with older people I was delighted to find Alex Comfort's book *A Good Age* (1977), which has dozens of portraits of people of all races who achieved great things in their old age. I copied some of these, mounted them on a board and wrote underneath something I had heard Professor Millard say, 'Old Age is not a Problem, it is an Achievement'. This was a very obvious way of using pictures to get a message across and it had the desired effect of provoking a lot of discussion and interest amongst residents, staff and visitors.

But while all pictures have a message of some sort, and usually different ones for different people, the pictures we buy to hang on the wall are to look at. So it is especially important that we select pictures which come from a wide variety of cultures and reflect that variety in their subject matter. It is important that when a person of African or Chinese or Indian descent walks into a residential centre, they see signs that their culture, race or nationality are respected and valued attributes, and are in some way recognised and part of the varied culture of the place. It is no less important that residents are supported and encouraged in their interest in and valuing of their own and other people's cultures, and have an expectation that they will live in a culturally rich and diverse environment.

INCLUSION/EXCLUSION

Acceptance

A fundamental message for residential homes to communicate is acceptance, respect and value for all individuals. (I use 'acceptance' in an active sense: see Beedell 1970.) One of the clearest ways in which we can do that is by looking at the messages we give in the pictures and images we choose. I do not mean that when you are visited by an Indian senior citizen with a view to taking up residence, you should rush out and buy some Bombay Mix and a take-away, put some sitar music on the tape machine and light some joss sticks; your visitor may care for none of these things, and she is very likely to know that her race and culture are not in any way part of normal life in this home. No, if we are genuinely attempting to make our services, wherever they are, open to all potential users in a multicultural and multiracial country (as Britain is) then we must start making the homes themselves reflect the diversity and richness of our culture before we can expect to establish the sort of atmosphere and environment in which all people can feel at home.

A residential home can be a place for new experience and knowledge, new friends and understanding; a place to try food you have never eaten before; to move to music you have never heard before; or to enjoy a celebration you have never known of before. What a chance, what an opportunity!

As workers we need to cultivate the skill of seeing the building, its contents and environment anew, each time we walk in. And we need to ask other people – residents, family, friends, social workers, people who have come to lay a carpet or fix the boiler – what do they see?

Public building or home; boundaries and doors; public and private space

We should think, 'What does this building, this room, this piece of equipment, say? Does this aspect of the building serve to include or exclude?' (See Appendix 3, Models, Images, Cultures.) Think about the entrance: what does it say to people who arrive or say about people as they leave the building? What sort of impression do you wish to convey? A home, like any other in the street? A public building? A block of flats? Or a special sort of home – a 'home'? A sanctuary? A safe place? A warm and friendly and welcoming place?

Some residential centres are too big and too obviously purpose-built to be disguised. (See also Chapter 8 for discussion of multipurpose social service centres.) In any case, why do we feel the need to disguise residential homes? A small, family-group home should be just that: a house where a small group of people live, not immediately identifiable as a 'home'. But a large residential home with twenty or more residents and a day centre attached is never going to look like a family home, and there is no sense in pretending that it is. Within it, however, we should aim to achieve an atmosphere of the essential elements of comfort, individuality and choice which we all want in our own home, our living space. So although the building is large and institutional, there are parts of it which are small, intimate and which express individuality and privacy; there are areas which are genuinely home to individuals and small groups.

The entrance to a large, busy, residential centre which includes a whole range of services will be a reception area, not simply a front door in the way a house or flat has a front door. This area is likely to be staffed in some way, by paid staff, residents, or volunteers whose job it will be to give information, direct people to other more private areas of the building or areas where public events are taking place, and occasionally to provide some security by restricting the entry of unwelcome visitors.

Visitors will experience the private nature of the living spaces in the centre when they get to them. To establish these distinctive differences in public and private space, staff and residents need to be quite clear about who goes where and the meaning of doors in the place. The door to a small group-living area will be that group's front door, under their control. If other staff (including managers), residents and visitors, fail to respect this boundary they will quickly render it and the sense of ownership, control and privacy engendered by it, meaningless. Residents' rooms, most obviously, are their private living spaces and, irrespective of whether the resident chooses to use the lock to the door, she or he should be in control of who goes into the room and when.

Kitchens, bathrooms and lavatories

When designing kitchens, laundries and bathrooms, we need the same awareness of public and private space, domestic or industrial use. A kitchen catering for large numbers of people must have suitable pieces of equipment for the job, and they will not be anything like the cookers, fridges and sinks found in ordinary household kitchens. Nor will the kitchen be suitable for use by residents and care staff although, occasionally, arrangements could be made for them to use it outside normal catering hours. There is no point in pretending that such a kitchen is a nice homely 'sitting around, cup of tea, and chat' sort of place. It isn't and it must not be, because its efficiency and ability to produce large quantities of high quality meals would be impaired.

But every *home* needs a kitchen, bathroom and lavatory which looks and feels homely. So, in large establishments where one or several of these rooms are institutional, we must think about how to provide others which are not and can be a living, integrated part of ordinary life. These rooms will be equipped with domestic items and will have the personal bits and bobs of everyday life around.

Although a bathroom may need a hoist installed for people who cannot get in and out of the bath without it, this does not mean that the rest of the room should look like a laboratory or clinic. This is a place to relax, to enjoy yourself, to be personal in very personal and comfortable surroundings. The same goes for lavatories which should be warm, private and welcoming and, of course, clean.

Taking a pride in the place

The physical fabric of the place will communicate its task, perhaps sooner and more clearly than any other aspect of its organisation. Undoubtedly, the ineffectual effort to disguise large establishments stems from our shame about how they are run. We do not try to disguise a school or a library or a hospital; indeed we try to make clear their purpose and social use. There is no shame in using or working in such institutions. Why are we then so ashamed of residential homes? We have taken part in a long process of derogation and disparagement which has afflicted and still afflicts residential care. Our task in creating helpful organisation is to create a place and do a job we are proud of and which we do not feel the need to shut away and hide.

Similarly, residents and their families, neighbours and the owning or managing organisations could be proud of their residential homes. They would be good places in which to live and work (see Chapters 7 and 8).

It is clear that different residential establishments and homes have different tasks and that in creating the basic provision, the fabric and the physical arrangements of the place, each establishment should seek to communicate its particular task.

FOOD AND CATERING

Food is another basic need which conveys immense symbolic meaning as well as being essential to physical survival. Food always matters: its quality, presentation, origins, its preparation, quantity and supply, as do the conditions we eat in, the cutlery and crockery we use and the company we eat with.

Let me start with the basics – providing good food which residents enjoy and eat and meals to look forward to.

Achieving these is no mean feat. Cooking and other aspects of catering are always bedevilled by the deeper meanings of the process. Even in places where the caterers do not have constant direct contact with the customers, the creative and stressful job of cooking can provoke shocking outbursts of anger and abuse. To have someone complain about a meal which has cost you so much in thought, time and effort can be devastating.

Some residents will not have had many good experiences of food. Quite typically, feeding as a baby may have been surrounded by problems. In addition, poverty and related living conditions may have meant that nourishing meals were hard to come by, and what food was available had to be competed for and eaten standing up or walking around. Many other residents will have experienced good food and feeding, and have internalised the experience as they took in the food as being good and nourishing. They will be expecting similar emotional and physical nourishment from the food in the home.

Either way, the food is unlikely to be what residents expect or are used to. Those who do not trust food and may have eaten a very limited and poor diet will be anxious and – oddly – scornful of anything new. They may suspect what to anyone else is obviously wholesome and nourishing food. And those with good experience of food and eating will be looking for the home cooking they are used to. The home's particular brand of home cooking will not satisfy them.

It is rare to encounter an enthusiastic and optimistic cook. They have suffered too much rejection and abuse; they tend to withdraw and become rather cynical to protect themselves against the criticism they have learned to expect. But the catering staff are at least as important as any other staff in the home. They must be given the status, respect and support to enable them to enjoy their very difficult work. Praise and appreciation for one good meal goes into the creative energy needed to produce the next good meal. But, much more frequently and easily, cooks receive criticism and indifference which leads to a downward spiral of performance.

Food, choice and culture

There must be choice in food and there must be diversity. Residents' physical and spiritual wellbeing will depend upon the nourishment provided by good food.

Even in organisations which claim to provide a multicultural service it is extremely rare to find a genuine choice – and I don't mean between roast beef with Yorkshire pud and a ham or cheese salad! We must think quite as much about the minority of residents as we do about the majority. We must also cater for minorities in the population who are excluded from using residential services because we do not routinely provide a choice of meals which are acceptable to them. In several settings where a long-established multiethnic choice of food has been available, residents or day attenders have shown increasing willingness and interest in trying new foods. It is worth reflecting that a very large proportion of English and British foods now regarded as traditional were once new to the indigenous population. We (the British) often display a shocking ignorance and prejudice (and deprive ourselves) when we will happily eat an ordinary banana and won't even try plantain or green banana.

Food is so much more than physical nourishment; it is at the heart of culture. Food is a part of all religions. Our beliefs affect the food we eat and how we prepare and eat it. Food affects our daily, weekly, monthly and yearly patterns of life, and our cultural events, celebrations and rituals. We get to know people when we eat with them. There is no more powerful message of acceptance, no better way of caring and communicating than to eat together.

We cannot adequately care for a person unless we provide the food they like and which can sustain their body and soul. Doing this is one of the most important but elusive parts of creating good residential care.

All staff concerned with the provision of residential care should read *More than Rice and Peas* by Sara Hill (1990). This is an inspiring and immensely informative book which makes clear connections between food and culture, history and patterns of everyday life – and with the racism which underlies the repeated failure to provide good food for all.

STAFF ORGANISATION

The way staff organise and conduct themselves carries another powerful message. In a home which proclaims that residents are encouraged and expected to take part in all the major decisions, it is ludicrous and deceitful to hear and see staff being treated in a disparaging and patronising way by managers. If hierarchical and domineering systems and practices are accepted as the fundamental path of staff relationships, inevitably the same will be true for relationships with and between residents.

Residential work is particularly prone to hierarchies, both formal and informal. If we wish to regard and treat residents as equal human beings (and there is no legitimacy in any alternative intention), we have to work hard at the same equality of regard between staff. The manager (see Chapter 4) will set the tone and will take care to spend time with staff and residents, to eat with them, to use the same lavatories and be subject to the same standards of behaviour from timekeeping to respecting personal boundaries.

Everything we do as members of a staff team will impinge on the residents. Our meetings, supervision and joint working on shifts will provide a model and a strong guide to the possibilities and potential for residents. When we have a disagreement, how do we sort it out? When someone is in trouble, what sort of advice and support do they get? Do we encourage each other to be assertive and self-directed? How do we work cooperatively together? How do we manage our meetings?

Staff meetings

The business of achieving effective team organisation is a constant struggle and is never completed. The principal forum for this work is the staff meeting.

Most places will need a staff meeting weekly. Although some people may need to be with residents during the meeting, everyone else should be able to attend. If it is not possible to get everyone on duty (paid) for a staff meeting once a week, the establishment is short staffed and cannot be expected to do an adequate job for users.

(Since the majority of establishments still do not have a frequent and regular staff meeting, and most organisations responsible for providing residential care do not provide sufficient staffing for them to do so, most residential homes cannot claim to be achieving one of the essential ingredients of a good service. Nor are most arms-length inspectors yet picking this failure up and demanding action.)

In a large establishment, small team meetings may alternate with the full staff meetings. Many of the principles of work and care will be practised at the meetings; for instance, in a place which is aiming to share responsibilities and where staff and residents are constantly given opportunities to develop their talents, where better to practise those principles than in the staff meeting? So, the formal roles in the meeting will be taken in turn: the chairing and minuting. A regular time and format is desirable, enabling everyone to take part and to know the possibilities and limitations of such a meeting.

Example 5.4   A purposeful network of meetings

At Inglewood we established a purposeful and sophisticated network of meetings.

On a Monday afternoon the management team had a business meeting. All the managers and team leaders were on duty. We took turns to chair and minute the meeting; the minutes were made available to all other staff and residents. The meetings were open for other staff and residents to attend if they wished. We followed this meeting with a team development group run by one of us or someone from outside.

On Tuesday afternoons we alternated the large staff meeting with the small team meetings for each unit. The large meeting (sometimes fifty people) included everyone who worked in the place and was again open to residents. The formal roles of chair and minute-taker were rotated. The meetings always started with the minutes of the previous meeting followed by reports from all the teams, including the management team and catering team; sometimes residents made reports on events that they had been involved in arranging. Each report was acknowledged by everyone clapping – a tradition which started spontaneously with the first report at the first such meeting. (The clapping was a loud and physically expressed sign of sharing our enthusiasm, pride and joint endeavour.)

The agenda was assembled in the previous week and anyone or any group could put an item down for discussion or decision. It was the chair's final decision about which items were discussed and in what order.

The meeting lasted up to one and a half hours and almost never overran its time. We arranged the seating in a large oval in our most spacious room, with the chair and minute-taker sitting at a table at one end.

The meeting was big and needed considerable structure to help it to be effective. It was a very important fortnightly event which was designed to keep a large and disparate staff group together, sharing values and a common vision, communicating with each other and experiencing joint progress. Everything was fed back to and then was given further impetus by the staff meeting.

It is important to draw attention to this illustration of the use of agreed procedures. Cooperation, participation and democracy are strengthened by adherence to good, simple procedural practice which legitimises and opens up decision making. The 'pseudo-democratic' style referred to in Chapter 4, p. 76 has none of this self-managed, internal discipline.

Example 5.4   (continued)

In addition there were many other meetings which regularly took place: individual supervision for all staff (including domestic workers), group workers' meetings, carers' support groups, residents' committees and a working group for just about everything that was ever planned and put into practice.

The practice of meeting, discussing and making decisions was led and modelled at the large staff meeting and the management meeting. Everyone in the place had experience of taking part in meetings and being able to make their voice heard; most people at some time had chaired or minuted meetings. Effective meetings were part of the culture and experience of the place from which much of the creativity and innovation sprang.

Checklist for staff meetings

* *Regular* – at least once a fortnight, same day, same time, same place. Start and finish on time. One and a half hours is long enough.
* *A central part of the work* – everyone rostered to be on duty.
* *Layout* – arrange room to help communication.
* *Procedure* – establish a simple order for doing things.
* *Agenda* – open to everyone to contribute.
* *Chairing and minuting* – rotate these jobs and make them formal.
* *Record discussions and decisions* – define action to be taken and name who is to take it.
* *Review* the decisions and subsequent action from the last meeting before deciding on further action.
* *Open* the meeting to residents wherever possible and encourage participation.
* *Protect* the meeting from outside interruptions but delegate staff (in turn) to attend to residents' needs during meeting.
* *Persevere* with meetings – don't give up when they are difficult or get stuck. Find ways to improve them – together.
* *The manager* should make attendance at the staff meeting a priority. If she misses them, the meetings will start to fall apart – and then so will the whole place!

SUPERVISION

Throughout this book there have been references to supervision. It is an unfortunate habit in social services work, and in residential work in particular, to discuss supervision as if everyone knows what is meant by the term and as if everyone received it. They don't – and they don't!

There are several excellent books on the subject and this part of this book is no substitute for reading one or more of these, nor is it a substitute for taking one of the many short courses in supervision which are available. I particularly recommend Atherton (1986), Hawkins and Shohet (1989), and Houston (1990) who have all contributed to my own theory and practice of supervision. However, equally, a lack of training and knowledge about supervision is not a reason not to get supervision (your own and other people's) started. Practising, as a supervisee and as a supervisor, will always be your principal means of learning how to do it.

I have long experience of supervision but I also have considerable experience of neither giving nor receiving it. In some of my stories and examples of residential work, I have mentioned my supervision or lack of it, how sometimes it was my nourishment for survival and how, at other times, I had to make do without. At some of those times when I had no regular supervision, for example, when I was missing the doctors' and dentists' appointments (See Chapter 2), my developing capacity to reflect on my own behaviour and to try to understand my motivation and unconscious processes was a sort of self-supervision. Similarly, sitting and writing a diary, or the process of mulling over an incident or even reading about the work you do (as at this moment) all have some of the essential elements of the supervisory process in them. To a limited, but very useful extent you can do some of your own supervision. Certainly by these thoughtful and reflective processes, away from the immediacy of the work situation, you are preparing yourself to use supervision and eventually to give it to someone else.

What is supervision? Gaie Houston (1990) writes of a person she is about to supervise who says that what she wants is 'SUPER vision'. She (the supervisee) expects through the process of supervision to be able to look at her work in a new – broad and deep – perspective. Later, Houston sums up what she thinks are the essentials of that process: for the supervisee to be

Held, listened to, encouraged;
Challenged, confronted, stimulated;
Disciplined, informed, answerable.

That is an excellent list which encompasses the wide range of activity and process in good supervision.

All of us know that we need space in which to talk about, reflect on and understand what we are doing and feeling. I have demonstrated what a difficult and demanding job residential work is; you will know this from acknowledging your own experience, not only from reading this and other books.

As workers and managers of our work, we are obliged to find some way of providing this reflective and learning space for ourselves and other people. This is supervision.

We have perpetuated many myths about this process: that it can be done only by a trained supervisor (whoever that is), that it takes only one form (usually individual, one-to-one meetings), that it is either strictly a managerial or non-managerial process. Many staff groups and managers talk about the need for supervision, and at the same time are expecting some sort of special extra input before it can be started. The extra input is not forthcoming and so it is never started. Often staff will go on supervision courses and return with a particular model which is impossible to institute in their work setting. This has a demoralising effect. My advice is to go on a course only if you are determined to put your learning into effect, to adapt what you have learned, to make a start on really finding out about supervision by *doing it*.

Starting supervision

All residential work jobs should now have a formal statement of your right and obligation to be supervised, and all management jobs should state your responsibility to give supervision. If you are not receiving supervision you may regard this as seriously as not receiving your pay. Make a fuss and don't take No for an answer.

Begin by acknowledging your need and the urgency of meeting that need in respect of continuing to work at an emotionally and intellectually demanding level. Within a couple of weeks of recognising your need, arrange to meet a supervisor. Who?

You should have a designated supervisor so you may ask for a meeting with that person. If not (or possibly in addition), consider the range of choices you have for someone to meet with: a colleague, a manager, a small group of staff or colleagues from several different settings, a friend in the same or similar work or a paid outsider who gives supervision as part of her work. Meet with them and work out a simple agreement which at least spells out times and dates, place, duration, limits of confidentiality, a clear statement of what you want from the sessions and a time to review what you are doing.

By using this advice and increasingly engaging in and learning from the process itself, by reading more detailed and fundamental discussions of supervision and perhaps by starting your own training, you will quickly become a competent supervisee. This practice and learning will then fit you, again quite quickly, to start giving supervision to other people.

Some useful tips for supervisors
* Provide a quiet and protected place – no phone, no interrupters.
* Supervision is not a 'chat' and cannot be done in the pub.
* Be there on time every time and finish on time.
* Be clear whose time this is – the supervisee's – and do not produce your own material.
* Your job is to listen more that it is to talk.

* Remember this process is to help the supervisee to do her/his job; it is not personal therapy.
* you are a second pair of ears and eyes, and a second brain and heart; use them to hear and see, think and feel and offer the resulting insights, observations, hunches and reactions to the person you are working with.
* Remember Gaie Houston's definition (p. 106)

If you are a manager in residential work you have the same responsibility to give and receive supervision as other staff, but you also are clearly more responsible for establishing the climate of support, learning and development for staff in which supervision will play a leading part. You will have to make sure that all staff are supervised regularly, that time and room are made available and that appropriate records are kept. Supervision is not an optional extra, nor should it be a spare-time, unpaid activity.

Staff support groups

Closely allied to supervision and the reasons for it are staff support groups. The purpose of such groups is to enable workers to work better and to create collective support, understanding and strength to apply to the job in hand. The groups may take various forms: a fortnightly session with an outside consultant or facilitator (see Chapter 9), women's groups, Black workers' groups, gay and lesbian workers' groups, groups formed around some specialist work or interest or working groups developing some particular project or event. Some may be regular and permanent with the remit of attending to staff communication and working relationships; others will run for a limited number of sessions tied to the felt needs of particular groups. Of course, you will always need to demonstrate a clear connection with and benefit for an improved service for residents.

These groups will be aimed at improvement and maintenance of care through the support and development of staff. Supervision, as we have seen, also has this role; indeed, meetings with these groups may sometimes be an alternative form of supervision. For example, group work is often best supervised in a group, so five workers who are leading various sorts of groups in a home may wish to have specific group work supervision from an outside consultant. Or they may simply meet regularly to review and discuss their work and act as supervisory consultants to each other.

Again there is a managerial responsibility to provide the time and space for these groups to work, and to have a regular oversight of their work. The group members will be responsible for reviewing their own progress and reporting on their use of the time.

TRAINING AND DEVELOPMENT

Some establishments have a very obvious training and development culture. As soon as you enter them there is evidence that staff are learning and changing. There is a notice board which advertises training events both inside and outside the place. At staff meetings training is discussed. All work is made part of the overall development of practice and it is clear that staff want to improve and advance their own individual work and the work of the whole place. Training events take place regularly; staff ask for training. Those who are not qualified aspire to receiving professional training and qualification. Domestic staff participate and are welcomed into this training culture – and so are residents and even their families and carers. Staff from other establishments come to events; everyone is encouraged to offer their experience and learn together. Students vie for placements at such establishments and are expected to contribute as much as they gain and, of course, gain by contributing.

Whether you are a manager or not, you have a right to training and professional development, and you have a responsibility to ask for training and to participate in the development of the team you work with.

Example 5.5   A training and development culture

One of the cooks does not know much about Caribbean food and cookery. There are two Jamaican residents at the home she works in and they are not getting food which they are used to or like. There has been a lot of discussion in staff meetings recently about how to provide a service which is welcoming and helpful to Black users. There is a growing awareness in the staff group that although there are a lot of Black staff, all other aspects of the place tend to give the message that it is suitable only for White residents. Staff go away from the last meeting with a remit to discuss and come up with proposals for ways to improve the service in their own units and areas of work.

The cook discusses this with her supervisor, an assistant manager, in their next meeting. She trusts her supervisor sufficiently to begin by talking about her initial resentment and her resistance to the idea that the food she was preparing was not good enough for the two Jamaican residents. She is able to talk about some of her attitudes and prejudices, and how low she feels when people criticise her cooking. Her supervisor, who is Black, listens carefully and with some relief.

The cook then says she wants to do something about it but doesn't know where to begin. Between them they think about all the resources both within the home and in the local area. The cook begins to realise that she does know quite a bit more than she thought. She lives locally, has Jamaican and other Caribbean friends and colleagues; she shops in the market and she is actually very interested in food.

Her supervisor has a professional connection with a local voluntary group which runs a luncheon club for Black pensioners. She also has books and recipes which she is willing to lend. She skilfully works with her supervisee, without overloading her with information nor telling her how to do it. The cook keeps her initiative and gets her supervisor's support and guidance.

Between them, using two supervision sessions, they create a training and development plan, initially centred on the cook but later including other staff. It goes something like this:

Research work: identifying foods available in the market; talking with other staff and the two residents about possible menus; reading – including something about the history and varied cultures of Caribbean food.
Training: five days at the luncheon club learning some of the basics of preparation, cooking and menu planning.
Planning and budgeting: in consultation with residents and staff preparing a menu to include a daily Caribbean dish; adjusting the use of the budget to accommodate buying suitable food.
Implementation: doing it! producing the new food.
Feedback and review: asking residents and staff for their opinion of the new menu and the meals themselves, and recording the results; introducing the plan at the next staff meeting and reporting back on progress each week; reviewing the plan and its implementation at supervision meetings.

The cook posted a copy of her plan on the staff training and development notice board for all to see. A lot of staff were willing to help and support her. The other cook, who was Spanish, was encouraged to prepare more food of her own culture and discovered common elements with some Caribbean dishes. She later initiated a similar training and development programme for herself, learning how to cook some Bengali snacks and meals which were added to the afternoon and evening menus.

These individual initiatives, combined with development work which other workers and teams were doing, led to great changes. The home was transformed: good, new smells came from the kitchen and visitors would enquire, 'What's cooking?' The production of each week's menu was of great interest to nearly everyone there, staff and residents. Meals were looked forward to, enjoyed and were a constant source of conversation. People sat around at meal times and an increasing number of local pensioners signed up for the luncheon club and for evening social events. And more Black pensioners started to come in, as visitors and as residents. The message was clear: there was a service here for them; they were welcome, not an awkward embarrassment.

As you may imagine, a culture of training and development which would enable these changes to occur itself takes planning and time to establish. The manager of the home is often most influential in creating such an atmosphere initially. She needs to be an enthusiast about training and to have experienced her own good training as well as being a trainer. Managers are trainers; it is part of their job. They must constantly give a high priority to training and to think about it in its widest sense. They must promote staff development in all areas of activity and at all levels. All staff have something to offer and much to gain, and this developmental culture is not confined to staff; residents too, of whatever age, should be given the opportunity to learn and to contribute to other people's learning.

ROTAS

Everything that has been written in this book so far – all the accounts of work, every mention of staff, their actions and responsibilities, and particularly my discussion in this chapter of staff organisation – depends on one central tool of helpful organisation: the rota. How can you get a staff group of seven, or twenty, or fifty doing all these things *and* providing the care, the steady, reliable and consistent attention to the needs of residents both as individuals and groups? It is a very tall order.

A good rota matches available staff resources to residents' needs. Its complexity is dictated very largely by the size of the workforce but obviously it must be comprehensible to staff and residents. Most rotas do not sufficiently meet residents' needs and are either far too mechanistic or are put together day by day or week by week, according to constantly changing circumstances.

A rota should be longterm and predictable. Workers need to be able to plan time off and time for important personal matters as well as their time with residents and for other business within the home. Residents, of course, need to be in a position to do exactly the same and, assuming staff are of importance to their lives, it is essential for them to know when individual people are going to be working.

In my experience there are no simple solutions to the construction of good rotas. Early/late patterns and splitting the staff into shift teams who always work together are likely quickly to develop competitive, divisive and defensive trends (see Chapter 6). If rotas are going to meet residents' needs above all others (but not to the exclusion of all others) then the rota has to be quite complicated and is likely to have a pattern which is of three weeks duration at the very least.

Constructing a rota

Staffing levels

Staffing numbers go up and down and it is unlikely that any place will be fully staffed all the time. Of course, the staffing establishment should take account of this (but rarely does). In very rough figures you will need four workers in post to provide one person on duty during the day (morning till night).

If the organisation's expectation is for there to be two staff on duty at all times during the waking day in a small home (or a unit of a larger establishment) then there must be a staff team of eight staff. Any less than seven people (full-time equivalent) will incur regular overtime or getting temporary staff to fill in.

So, first:

Check your staffing levels to see if they can give the care your organisation is purporting to provide.

If they cannot, immediately register your demands, backed up by figures.

(There are several, more precise methods of calculating staffing requirements; still one of the best is described in *Staffing in Residential Homes*, Social Care Association 1980.)

What should the rota provide?

Make a list of your essential requirements of the staff team. This may look something like this for daytime staffing of a small home:

* Two people on duty at all times of the waking day.
* One person to 'sleep in on call' each night and this person to be working the night before and the morning after.
* All staff on duty for the staff meeting (weekly).

* 'Hand-over' of at least half an hour when shifts overlap.
* A consistent pattern of working for all staff.
* Identification of the person who is coordinator for each shift (duty person).
* Every team member should work with every other team member at some point in the rota.
* Time allowed for training, supervision and staff development.
* Time built in for record keeping, outside contacts and visits, phone calls, etc. (If you do not build in this time, staff will have to use that which is intended for direct work with residents – which should always be the largest proportion of their time.)
* Senior staff should all be on a publicly displayed rota, with everyone else, and should be accountable to colleagues and residents for how they spend their time.
* Everyone should get a roughly equal amount of prime time off (weekends, evenings, etc).
* In most situations you will need to consider the balance of staff on duty – seniority, women and men.

(Every extra requirement you add will complicate the construction of a suitable rota.)

The requirements and constraints of the rota should be discussed with staff and residents but it is not usually possible to construct a rota in committee. I have found that it takes several hours with paper, pencil (and rubber!) to come up with a draft rota to put before the team for discussion and comment. It then takes further work to incorporate what you can of the feedback. (I have not tried using a computer to construct a rota but I imagine this could be a great help. However, I would be very wary of programmes which purported to produce rotas to order unless, as is quite possible, they included all the variables such as those listed above.)

No rota can satisfy everyone or every requirement. It is always a compromise and becomes better with use and fine adjustment. To work well, a rota has to be owned and supported by the staff team as a whole. Staff can sabotage a rota quite quickly by swapping shifts and by avoiding unpopular shifts.

It is quite common for outside managers in organisations to invent and then impose a universal or standard rota for all residential establishments of the same sort. This is always a failure; it is not their job and it displays an ignorance and total misconception of the residential management task.

As can be seen from the very basic list above of suggested requirements for the rota, these will vary from one establishment to another; all residential homes and their residents and workers are different, with different needs and priorities at different times. The responsibility for deploying the staff resources to their optimum effectiveness for residents lies with the staff of the home, not with a detached and remote outsider. Of course, not all outside managers are detached and remote but the act of inventing and imposing a rota, rather than helping the staff to produce one themselves, implies unsound and distant management.

ROUTINES, RULES AND HABITS

Residential homes are prone to the growth of routines which are not helpful to residents. Life becomes very ordered and dull, and staff and residents can be at the mercy of an unchanging, unimaginative routine. (This institutionalising tendency and our capacity to resist it are discussed in the next chapter.)

However, most of us use routine as a very personal and important way of managing our lives. I get up at roughly the same time each morning, make tea, wash, dress, go out and buy the paper, have breakfast and read the paper while others in my household are going through their own routines This has not always been my habit and it is likely to be changed many times in the future, but it is important to me now while the circumstances of my working life are varied and uncertain. If my work patterns were more predictable I might well be less attached to – even willing to relinquish – the sustaining regularity of my present morning routine.

The same situation will apply to many other people. We construct our routines to help with the complicated business of managing life. They can however be obsessive and defensive so that instead of enabling other things to happen they become blocks to change and development. (Again, more will be said about such defences in Chapter 6.)

We have seen how children can use a routine (Chapter 3, Bedtime p. 52), a particular regular order of doing things, to manage getting up or going to bed. Their routine of having supper, a piggy-back upstairs, cleaning their teeth, going to the lavatory, listening to a story, being tucked up and kissed goodnight, wanting the exact words repeated when we say goodnight and the ones they say back, the door being left open just the right amount, the landing light being left on, the last minute check of who is on duty in the morning and 'Will my jeans be ready?' This is a routine with ritual elements which have been constructed by the child to meet precise and real needs. We agree to the routine; we use it to meet those needs. At an appropriate time, signalled by the child or sometimes prompted by us, we may start trying to leave out parts of the routine, or do other things. Typically, the supper ritual might change or we don't need to be told when a piggy-back is no longer right for this child, or that she now wants the door closed and will read for a while before going to sleep. But it will have been partly by using the routine that the child has been able to move on.

We tend to caricature older people by their habitual behaviour, and label routinised behaviour as especially typical of old age. But like anyone else's, older people's routines are often a practical and reasoned response to circumstances, and sometimes are an emotional anchor to help them to manage a very uncertain or threatening world. It follows that moving into and living in a residential home will be a time to establish new and helpful routines as well as to hang on to some old ones.

Routines are most likely to be evident around the ordinary everyday business of life, getting up, going to bed, preparing food and drinks, eating, sleeping, emptying bowels and bladder, and activities such as reading the paper, watching television, meeting people, shopping and keeping in touch.

This points to the importance of supporting people's individual routines and creating an environment in which those important, personal, small rituals can both continue and, if and when necessary, be let go of. We should remember that many of these habits are of fundamental cultural or religious significance. Watching *Neighbours*, *Coronation Street* or *Top of the Pops*, however incomprehensible their importance may be to some people, may be extremely important to the resident. (I don't like to miss *The Archers*!) Washing before a meal, or saying a prayer, eating in a certain way or order, fasting or giving up meat can be dismissed as fussy and trivial but are usually major statements and commitments.

Habits and agreements, not rules and contracts

Most of us will have come across organisations, particularly residential centres, in which it is stated that there are hardly any rules. Residents may be told, 'We have only two rules here: tell us when you are going out and no smoking in bedrooms.' The reasons for having rules are often attributed to some quasi-legal requirement outside the influence of the home's management; in the above case it would be the fire regulations. Usually we will discover quite quickly, whether we are staff or resident, that there are in fact a whole host of other rules as well; but they are not called rules.

In a place in which young people are detained and locked up, a place where residents do not *choose* to live, there are going to be rules, and, yes, they will be to some extent legally imposed from outside. It is vital that residents and staff here have a very clear, written list of these rules. But within these limitations it is especially important that residents (and by implication staff) learn how to manage their own lives and relationships better, and here the imposition of extra rules does not help. Nevertheless, there will be the need to establish good habits of social behaviour and make *agreements* between members of the community – a statement which largely sums up the importance of creating establishments that serve positive purposes, even though they house young people who have been judicially detained.

In the vast majority of residential settings which are non-custodial, it would be reasonable, even vital, to be told what the rules are before making the choice and commitment of going to live or work there. It may sometimes be necessary to remind residents (and staff) that the general framework of law applies to them as to everyone else. Assault is a prosecutable offence, whether committed in a residential home shared by five people who have some intellectual disability, or in a private household consisting of three children, two parents and an aged person who is suffering from Alzheimer's disease, or whether committed in the street. Wherever we live, we are subject to the law. It is our only recourse in situations which get out of hand, exceeding our capacity to sort things out by mutual negotiation and agreement.

But in a residential establishment, even a large one, in which people are living (and learning to live) together, there is no need to invent additional rules and operate them as if they were part of a special legal system with its own investigation procedures and its own enforcing punishments. Of course, we need to create a structure within which mutual negotiation and agreement are fostered (see Meetings, p. 103–5); but as soon as we start building a system of rules and regulations, sanctions and punishments, policies and procedures – our own, special and internal system of law – we are taking the road that leads to institutionalisation.

Often the signs of this insidious process can be seen in notices:
PLEASE WASH YOUR HANDS More suited to a public lavatory than to a toilet shared by a group of people living together as a household; STAFF ONLY Divisive – the 'them and us' attitude; THIS DOOR MUST BE KEPT LOCKED AT ALL TIMES Threat; punishment; 'keep out'; the 'lock-up' mentality.

And these printed notices, screwed to the door or wall, are reinforced by ubiquitous reminders, often scruffy, always bossy, telling you to wash your mugs, or leave the work area tidy, or warning that anyone found doing or not doing such and such will be – what? Taken from this place and hanged by the neck?

Of course it is a good habit to wash your hands after using the lavatory. But how did we learn it? Not, I suggest, from a notice over the handbasin. If we live with other people we have to learn to do our fair share of common household jobs; we need to know something about hygiene; we have to accept some responsibility for the security of the building. None of these things is ever completely learned or resolved. At home I do more than my fair share of some of the household jobs and less of others. We argue about it sometimes; I get scolded and I sometimes have a go at other people but we do not invent household laws, put up notices and levy fines for misbehaviour. We try to reach agreements and change our habits.

I believe everyone has the right to work out and learn, and go on learning, how to live socially, whether in a small or large group. Rules and set punishments are not the way we learn to live our ordinary life. Why, then, should they be regarded as an essential feature of institutional life?

Smoking

This is one of the most common causes of conflict in residential care. I select it for detailed discussion to illustrate the broad message that such social and communal issues cannot be successfully resolved by inventing and enforcing rules, but only by changing attitudes and relationships and learning to work at problems together.

Smoking is the source of much institutional 'legislation'. Typical rules in a children's home would be:

* Children are not allowed to smoke until they are 16 and then they may smoke only in designated areas of the house.
* Anyone under 16 caught smoking has the cigarettes taken away, is fined, and/or punished in some other way.
* Staff are allowed to smoke only in designated areas and at break times.

As all experience shows, when rules such as these are formulated nearly all the children and some of the staff will simply flout them or bend them in some way. Tensions between smoking and non-smoking staff will be rife and some smokers on the staff will collude with children, who will observe and internalise staff attitudes and behaviour. The gap between 'Do as I say' and 'Do as I do' will be wide. Staff and children will spend a good deal of their time on smoking-related matters, and the rules which are intended to deal with the problem will magnify it.

The inevitable consequence of the rule-based approach is that smoking becomes one of the most popular and subversive activities.

Cigarettes and places to smoke them gain a special institutional value. Around smoking there grows a powerful, attractive and probably violent subculture which is very like, and which may prepare young people to enter, illegal drug subcultures and lifestyles.

Such a system of rules is pointless, dangerous and irrelevant, and has no basis in law. As I understand it, the only law which relates directly to children and tobacco is that it is illegal for a shopkeeper to sell tobacco to anyone under sixteen. It can do no good, and it usually does much harm, to pretend that the internal smoking rules of a residential home have legal status.

General recognition that the traditional ways of tackling the smoking problem are at best ineffectual and at worst harmful should encourage us to look for a radically different approach. As the following example shows, an open and honest appraisal of attitudes and behaviour (by grown-ups and children alike) is the essential first step towards change.

Example 5.6   Getting to grips with a delinquent subculture

Having had little success with reducing the young people's smoking, and acknowledging the time and energy spent trying to police smoking in the fashion described above, the staff of a home for children and young people discuss a new approach at their weekly staff meeting.

First they face up to the situation they are in. Many of the residents have come to the home as regular and habitual smokers. Others quickly latch on to the illicit smoking culture and begin to smoke regularly. In this respect, coming to live in the home has damaged them, for some younger children who have experimented with smoking at the home would not have continued if doing so had not been so subculturally significant. They do not like smoking and yet continue to smoke. Smoking brings all these young people into conflict with the staff and 'the rules': conflict which can also be in some senses addictive and is certainly a way of avoiding other issues. Staff, too, become obsessed with smoking, the breaking of rules and the best way to punish children who do.

The staff now begin their discussion, starting from scratch. One practical step can be taken at once. It is illegal for shops to sell cigarettes to anyone under sixteen, so staff will be vigilant and firm about trying to stop those children from buying cigarettes. They will speak to shopkeepers known to be selling children cigarettes; if necessary, they will report them to the police for doing so. Recognising however that they can neither prevent children from buying cigarettes if they are really determined to do so nor invoke the law to tell them it is illegal for them to smoke, the staff resolve to make clear by their actions and attitudes that they *want* the children to stop. They do not invent rules or punishments to go with their intentions because they realise that it is they as staff who have to change before they can expect the young people to do so.

They discuss the example that they are setting to the children. They agree that there has been a lot of illicit smoking on their part and collusion with the children who smoke. Some staff have offered cigarettes to and accepted them from children. Some have smoked in the kitchen. The staff meeting is held in the main sitting room where children are not allowed to smoke, and yet smoking is permitted at the staff meeting. (Cigarettes are put out at that point in the discussion.) They have smoked in the staff sleeping-in room, when children are not allowed to smoke in their bedrooms. Some staff have even confiscated cigarettes from younger children and smoked them themselves; in effect they have stolen the children's cigarettes. It emerges that staff who have punished children for smoking have, in other circumstances, rewarded them with cigarettes. Some have displayed their own addiction to the children and boasted about the early age that they started smoking, thereby gaining, as they imagined, some 'street cred'!

As they examine their own delinquency honestly, they begin to understand how and why smoking is such an issue – for them, for the young people and for the place. They clearly have to start behaving differently. They need to control and manage themselves and their delinquency. No more boasting and lying, no more projection of badness, dishonesty and law-breaking on to the children. Some – not all – members of staff will be able to stop smoking altogether; in response to the children's enquiries they may say, 'I know it's bad for me and for you, but before I can expect you to give up, I must do so myself.' Smokers have invented thousands of ways of giving up the habit, and for a committed residential worker there can be few better ways than remembering that your bad example may be directly influencing a child with whom you work. Those who cannot give up altogether can at least stop smoking at work and thus avoid presenting the children with a bad example.

Having considered their own behaviour and how they can change it, the staff group are able to formulate their aim, which is to establish an anti-smoking culture in which the expectation – the thing to do – would be *not* to smoke. They want to create a new climate of opinion in which smoking is no longer a punishable offence, but an unfashionable and

unsociable activity. Because they have honestly appraised their own attitudes and conduct they are now in a position to consider how to enlist the
cooperation of others, the residents, visitors and colleagues who work in
other areas but come into the home on business. They agree together that
the following proposals are reasonable.

1 Most importantly, there would be no punishments for smoking (since
punishments have proved ineffectual and are, for some children, part of its
attraction). It would be recognised as a harmful and self-destructive habit.
Breaking the link between smoking and punishment would mean that in
this home smoking would no longer be automatically and seductively
associated with an illicit subculture and its attendant delinquency and
penalties.
2 All staff, that is, people employed in any way for the care of children and
young people, would be required not to smoke while working at or visiting
the home. All non-staff visitors would be asked not to smoke. (Like the
resident children, their parents, family and friends would find it possible to
smoke in some parts of the building but now more difficult in the changed
atmosphere.) In rooms in which smoking constituted an obvious health
hazard to others – the kitchen, dining room, main sitting room and office,
for example – everyone would be asked not to smoke. In other rooms,
anyone who wanted to smoke would be expected to ask whether people
minded and to respect their wishes if they objected.

Knowing that it would take a long time and the cooperation of the
residents to effect such a radical change in the life and culture of the home,
and accepting that changing their own attitudes and behaviour would not
happen overnight, staff thought it important to talk with the residents as
soon as possible. They resolved, therefore, to use the residents' meeting
that evening to tell them what they had discussed at the staff meeting and
to ask them to express their feelings and opinions.

The staff had a low expectation of the outcome, fearing a cynical
response: 'This is just another trick to catch us out and punish us.' They
recognised that their past record of dealing with smoking did not entitle
them to trust. They had spent many hours thinking up new ways of catching
children smoking and punishing them for it. However, it was agreed that
the four workers on duty that evening should tell residents what was
proposed.

In fact, they got a very different response when they reported the
discussion to the residents, candidly describing their own past attitudes to
the situation. Although some of the residents wished to retaliate, to return
some of the punishment which had been handed out to them, after a
surprisingly short period of expressing anger and resentment (which the
staff accepted) a few of the residents began to make constructive comments

and suggestions. They put forward their own ideas about which rooms should be non-smoking and about ways of cutting down or stopping their own smoking.

This particular staff meeting and decision, followed up as it was by the inclusion of residents in taking on and managing a destructive aspect of life in the home, proved to be a watershed. Smoking was drastically reduced, and many other things also began to change. As staff considered their individual attitudes and behaviour with regard to smoking, they recognised the wider implications of that particular issue. As they succeeded in bringing residents into their discussions and in enabling them to participate in decisions, they understood that smoking was but one of many areas of conflict rooted in a fundamentally flawed regime – ineffectually authoritarian and not cooperative.

Having successfully interrupted, and then reversed, a punitive 'us and them' spiral, the staff of that home were for ever afterwards suspicious of and resistant to inventing rules and punishments. From then on, they looked for meaningful connections between their own and the residents' behaviour. Residents' meetings were invested with growing importance and responsibility, leading to the establishment of the community meeting (non-smoking!) attended by everyone who lived or worked in the home, and recognised as its main discussion and decision-making meeting.

Rituals and celebrations

Rules, as we have seen, are institutionalising; they are externally imposed and are likely to become oppressive. They are measures taken to control people, to order their lives for them in a way which cannot then be taken in, internalised, to play a natural and integral part of a person's life. Rules become barriers to personal development. Yet we have also seen how individual routines and small rituals are important in managing one's life. They grow from within and only become a nuisance when they have outlived their use and a change is called for.

It is the same for groups and organisations. A group culture grows from the habits, small rituals and celebrations of a community. I have given many examples of this: the large staff meeting at Inglewood, the community meeting at Frogmore, establishing a training culture, supper and bedtime routines. All good residential homes have their rituals. However, we must be wary of group behaviour becoming ritualised (dominated by ritual) when the people serve the ritual rather than the other way round, so we must keep all such activity under stern and unsentimental review.

Birthdays are usually a good time for celebration, although we should always be careful to ask the person whose birthday it is how she or he would like to celebrate it, if at all. Certainly, leaving needs to be marked and acknowledged as an important event in the life of the home and in the life of the person who is leaving. This applies just as much to residents as it does to workers.

And death, above all, should be acknowledged and marked. Establishments where someone's death is virtually ignored and quickly forgotten are not fit to accommodate or work with people. In some homes, it seems as if once someone has died they never existed. By the next day their room is cleared and all trace of their life has been tidied away, parcelled up and disposed of. A fellow resident may say weeks later, 'Whatever happened to Tom? I haven't seen him for ages. Is he ill?' And it is quite possible that she is told, 'He's gone away'.

Death is hard to bear whether you liked the person or not. The ritual and process of dealing with the body, informing people, arranging the funeral and usually inviting friends and relatives to eat and drink together afterwards, are important ways of mourning, of accepting loss and saying goodbye, of recognising the worth of the dead person, of voicing and enacting some of our feelings. It is within these rituals that we can make contact with our feelings which may otherwise remain held in and unexpressed because there is no recognised time or place for them.

Each culture and religion has a different way of dealing with dying, death and mourning, and there are then many variations within cultures and religions. It is very important for all concerned that individual wishes and practices are allowed and accepted. For instance, in most Muslim cultures, no non-Muslim should touch the body after death, nor should the body be washed. Only men attend funerals. Women on the staff of a home could, however, pay their respects at the dead person's family home three days after the death. A priest (Brahmin) would visit a dying Hindu resident and would probably tie a thread around his or her wrist or neck. The dying person should be allowed to lie on the floor to be closer to the earth. If someone of the Jewish faith dies, it is likely that a relative will wish to sit with the body until the funeral (usually burial), which should take place within twenty-four hours.

Of course, it is not possible to know everything about every culture and religion or even about your own but a caring, valuing and accepting attitude is essential. To provide residential services well we must understand that religious and cultural rituals are of the deepest significance and meaning, and must never be treated as weird or outlandish because we have not come across them before.

Example 5.7   Religion and culture: bad practice

The family of a Muslim resident had explained to staff in a home that she needed to wash in running water (which could be water poured from a jug) before praying and after going to the toilet. The resident was very disabled and could not use the taps and basins, so she was reliant on staff bringing a jug and a basin for her to wash in.

One member of staff resented the small amount of extra thought and trouble involved in this, and questioned why the resident couldn't wash 'normally' like everyone else. She said she intended to treat her like the others but she would make a concession to 'their ways' by running down the corridor with the basin of water. In this way, she joked, the resident would be getting her 'running water'.

This chapter has covered a lot of ground but there is much that is left out. Creating helpful organisation is a complex, massive and unending task of which I have discussed what I consider to be the most important aspects. You may be surprised by what I have included and by the absence of such current 'essentials' as *care plan* and *keyworkers*. You will be able to find these subjects well covered elsewhere; indeed, nearly all writing on residential work makes them the central planks of organising practice. This and preceding chapters should help you to work out and apply the concepts of planning with residents and of staff taking personal and individual responsibility for implementing the plans. Both those closely related ways of working have been fundamental to good practice long before the widespread use of the new terms to describe them.

Whenever I encounter words and phrases, prescriptions and formulae which appear to have been swallowed whole by our profession, I want to ask fundamental questions. It is not a simple task to create helpful organisation in residential care and we should have learned by now that most of each decade's crop of new blueprints turn out to be failures or – worse – can be implemented as dominating and abusive practice. ('Pin-down' was just such a blueprint.) I ask myself what – if anything – the new phrases mean to residents, and I wonder what is the motivation behind setting up universal 'care planning' and 'keyworker systems'. Such questions will be explored in the next chapter.

Chapter 6

Resisting hindering organisation

ORGANISATION(S)

The word 'organisation(s)'is used here in three ways; the particular contents and arguments of this chapter make it desirable to define them.

1 ORGANISATION: the process of organising.
2 ORGANISATION(S): a place or institution (like a residential home) or a formation of people and groups which has a common and defined overall task (like a social services department or a voluntary society).
3 ORGANISATION: an established way of working or of conducting business, a complex construction of rules, procedures, guidelines and common practice which is created over time and is intended to help the achievement of the task in hand.

The use of each meaning is demonstrated in the following paragraph, and all three meanings are signified by the word as it is used in the chapter title.

Every organisation is a hindering one. Organisation which is consciously designed and constructed to help (see Chapter 5), quickly and unconsciously reconstructs itself to hinder. Managing residential work is essentially a process of constant renewal of helpful organisation and resistance to hindering organisation.

In this chapter I will consider how and why we so often end up organising *against* the task when we intend to do the very opposite, and how we can resist that process. I use two related ways of understanding organisation(s) which I have found useful as a manager and as a consultant:

1 The organisation as a 'socio-technical system' (Trist and Bamforth 1951; Rice 1958).

2 The propensity of organisations to construct systems which defend against the anxiety provoked by the primary task (Jaques 1955; Menzies 1970).

The primary task

Organisation is both the friend and the enemy of the primary task. While writing this book and constantly while working in residential care, I direct and discipline my thinking and my actions by using the idea of the *primary task*, that is the reason for the organisation's existence; the proper focus of its effort; the job without which it has no legitimate reason for functioning.

The definition of the primary task should be as simple and short as you can make it. For instance, a home for older people could define its task as 'To provide the accommodation and care which will meet the needs and choices of older people who cannot continue to get those needs and choices met in their own homes'. A privately owned home, a money-making business, may add 'To make x amount of money by providing accommodation and care, etc'. Having stated the primary task, it is then possible to test every action against the performance of the task. Anything which is not connected with achieving the primary task should be rejected.

Why do residential care establishments so often appear to fail in the performance of their primary task? How is it that homes which were built and staffed to meet the needs of residents end up as organisations which are geared to the needs of staff and management? A series of scandals, enquiries and prosecutions in private and council homes in the late 1980s and early 1990s have shown that things can go dangerously wrong.

ORGANISATIONS AS SYSTEMS

In his work on group processes, Bion (1968, 1980) introduced the idea of a primary task. He proposed that every group has a primary task but this task is not fixed or defined; it fluctuates according to the stages and performance of the group. Utilising this idea in relation to residential homes, as several writers have done before me, I need to have a more static, more directional definition of the primary task. And even if the group (whether staff and/or residents) begin to organise themselves and the place in a different direction, away from the stated primary task, they cannot, as Bion proposed, then constantly change the primary task. (Since Bion was – and I am now – discussing what are mostly unconscious

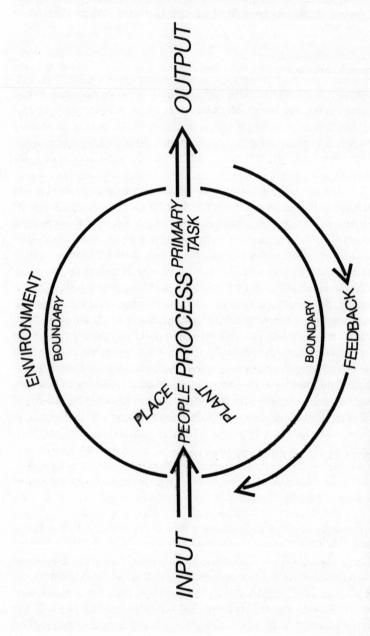

Figure 6.1 An organisation as a socio-technical system

processes, the act of identifying and defining any but the stated primary task is always done with hindsight.)

Socio-technical systems

To perform this task the organisation will require PEOPLE and PLANT, and a PLACE in which to do the job. The interaction of people and plant within the organisation to achieve the primary task we can call the PROCESS (Figure 6.1).

Around the organisation is a BOUNDARY, within which is the organisation and outside of which is its ENVIRONMENT. Goods, raw materials, supplies, water, electricity and gas, and all other intangible supplies which come into the organisation are the INPUTS, and all the things which come out of the organisation are OUTPUTS. This works both as a metaphor of organisation and at a literal level whether it be a small factory with raw materials going in, being processed (made into the product) by people and plant, and then going out again (output) and being sold, or whether it is a prison with inputs of prisoners, food, etc, a primary task of containment or rehabilitation and an output of ex-prisoners going back into the environment they came from. In both cases, the FEEDBACK loop is important to the definition of the primary task and how it is done. In the case of the factory, if the product does not sell, it may be the wrong thing, too expensive or badly made; if so, changes will have to be made to the primary task or the performance of it in order to keep this factory open. In the case of the prison, if prisoners escape (in the prison whose primary task is containment) or are being released and re-enter the environment unchanged by their experience in prison (the PROCESS), and reoffend only to come back again to prison, the feedback again demonstrates that the primary task is not being achieved or may be the wrong task altogether.

We can use this idea in residential work to think about our organisations – residential homes and the wider organisations of which they are part (Figure 6.2).

Defensive systems

Readers who have read from the beginning of this book and who have reflected on their own experience of working in residential care will know how fundamentally frightening and disturbing the work is. I have taken care to spell out the emotional hurt and dilemmas involved in getting close to people who are living in residential homes. We know they themselves have often been hurt and disturbed, and knowing what has happened to

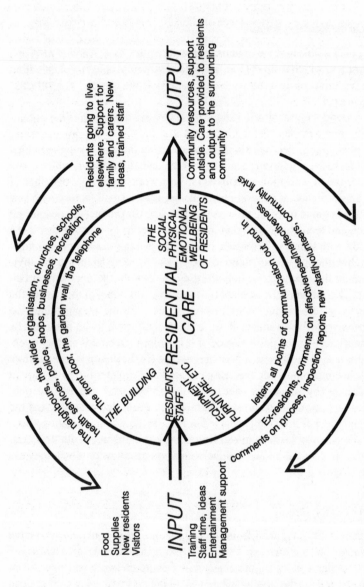

Figure 6.2 A residential home as a socio-technical system

people we are working with (think of a child who has been sexually abused) raises a confusing mixture of feelings in us.

Our proximity to other people's current pain will recall and rekindle our past and present experience of similar events and emotions. Working with someone who is dying, or very sick, or disabled is hard going – if we care about them. We need to protect ourselves from people who are very angry or violent, or perhaps even have some illness which they could pass on to us. We know that the negotiation of dependence and independence provokes great anxiety in carer and cared-for. We have seen how risky it is to get attached to clients and for them to get attached to us. We feel that making real and personal commitments and relationships is part of the job, essential to performing the primary task, and yet we are constantly told that we must detach ourselves.

I have discussed the ways in which we, individually, may withdraw or protect ourselves from the actual or potential harm which the work may do us, and how by doing so we may no longer be able to engage with the deepest and most pressing needs of residents. However, what Elliot Jaques (1955) and later Isobel Menzies (1970) have demonstrated is that these individual defences are matched and most powerfully backed up by unconscious organisational defences.

Goffman (1961) illustrated and analysed the process and effects of institutionalisation but he did not at that stage show exactly how that process is so necessary for the survival of staff in institutions when confronted by the pain, dependency and suffering of residents or patients.

Menzies demonstrates how the systems which originally were designed to further the task are hijacked to protect staff from the anxiety of attending to the task.

In Figure 6.3, illustrating a residential establishment as a hindering organisation, the PLACE, PEOPLE and PLANT become compartmentalised, separated from each other, and defended from the anxiety engendered by the PRIMARY TASK. The *integration* of the parts of the system in order to carry out the primary task (illustrated in Figure 6.2) has become *separation*.

All INPUTS are channelled into their designated area. New residents are subject to an admission procedure which is likely to be impersonal and is designed to communicate the institution's values and power to exert control.

The building, equipment and furniture bear few positive signs of people. It may be smart or vandalised but it won't be *personal*. (Graffiti can be a sign of desperate attempts to make personal marks on impersonal fabric.) Parts of the building and much of the furniture and equipment are

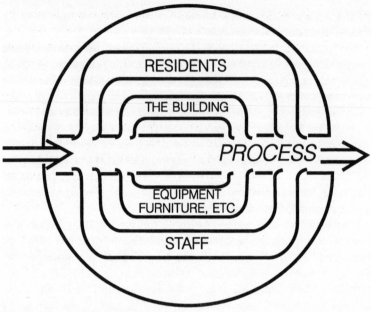

Figure 6.3   A hindering organisation

protected from or restricted to resident use. Locks and keys proliferate, under the exclusive control of staff.

Staff have a whole special and separate system to themselves of lavatories, staff rooms, crockery and cutlery, social activities, uniforms or an accepted convention about the way people dress. People have increasingly specialised jobs and complicated titles. The accomplishment of work has been systematized into a set of procedures and reduced to 'competences'. There may even be work sheets on which to record the completion of each step of the process.

Residents are in *their* areas – often called the 'unit', dressed in a uniform or in an accepted, conventional way. They have a system in the same way as the staff do. There is a hierarchy (pecking order) to match the staff's, and a separate set of rules and procedures.

The PROCESS of care is dignified and compartmentalised by names like 'programme', 'treatment plan', 'assessment', 'rehabilitation', or any word that denotes a planned, hard, defined and impersonal activity. It is very much a process in that it 'processes' people; it is done *to* people; it is likely to be detached from the ordinary living activities and human relationships – the areas of greatest risk – which are the very stuff of good residential care. Young people, for instance, are put through an 'independent living programme' (which is surely a contradiction in terms), and 'objective assessments' are made by the application of a series of tests and monitoring tools.

The primary task (to meet residents' needs) has virtually disappeared. It may occasionally be retrieved, groomed and trotted out to grace an Open Day, a fundraising activity, a committee report or a 'mission statement'. But engagement with the primary task has been prevented by the introduction of powerful defence systems of which such empty rhetoric as 'mission statements' are part.

Those readers who have experienced such institutions may find this description and brief analysis exaggerated and offensive. My example below will provide a more gradual and realistic explanation of how organisation designed to help very easily becomes defensive and hindering.

Example 6.1   The kitchen cupboard list

I remember in a children's home (Frogmore) the list on the back of the kitchen cupboard door which showed which jobs the staff should do on which days of the week. For instance: Mondays – laundry, packing, recording, despatching the dirty laundry and reversing the operation for the incoming clean laundry. Tuesdays – clean and tidy the kitchen cupboards and do the food order for the Co-op., etc. These jobs often didn't get done as they were meant to. Forgetting the laundry was a heinous crime and involved a lot of extra work for someone else. The subject was regularly brought up in staff meetings and new ways devised of getting these jobs done, some of which would work for a few weeks before falling into disrepair again and going through the same process of discussion and redesign.

All the jobs on that list were in some way disconnected from the children and young people in the place. Of course, food and laundry affected the residents but they were arranged in such a way that they became things for staff to do when the children were not there. The implication of our concentration on running the household, when at last we could do so without hindrance from the children, was that this was the real work of the place – when the children were absent. And we 'managed' these tasks by systematizing or inventing procedures to cope, thereby removing responsibility from the staff who were supposed simply to follow the procedure.

The written instructions also reduced our work to a step-by-step completion of a routine, simplifying and ordering quite basic tasks.

Our staff meetings became times at which staff were judged as good or bad, competent or incompetent, responsible or irresponsible, according to their performance of a set-down procedure (on the back of the kitchen cupboard door!). And we also spent most of our meetings talking about issues which were not 'child centred', not directly to do with the primary task.

I and some of my colleagues knew there was something wrong with all this and got very angry and frustrated by the seemingly circuitous and ineffective process.

Our responses were only partially helpful. I tore down the job rota and we decided that half of every staff meeting should be devoted to discussion centred on the children. However, what I did not understand at the time was that we were not simply dealing with aspects of institutionalisation as I knew of them, particularly from reading Goffman; we were confronting hidden and unconscious defences in which we had all colluded in building and maintaining in our organisation. This complex and sophisticated defence system was constructed to protect us from the task – the primary task – of directly engaging with and meeting the needs of the residents. These needs were so overwhelming, frightening and disturbing; they touched our own needs and emotions so painfully that we had to protect ourselves, individually, but, even more effectively, by a collective, collusive but unconscious defence system.

By not understanding that these defences existed in this way, our actions to deinstitutionalise our work and to become more child centred were partly ineffectual. Removing the jobs rota from the cupboard door did not remove the felt need for it. Some of my colleagues were furious with me and we then entered a long debate about the need for routines and order. I was categorised as 'anti-order', and I put them in a box marked 'institutionalised'. This did not help our communication but served as another layer of defence against the primary task and all it entailed.

Ten years later, at Inglewood, having analysed the process of change at Frogmore with the benefit of Isobel Menzies' work, I knew that simply attempting to demolish institutional practices will usually result in their reproduction elsewhere with a renewed tenacity. Such defences are hydra-headed. I had learned that the focus on the primary task, the capacity of staff to open themselves to the pain and feeling of the work, would come only through building an organisation which was specifically designed to support staff in doing a difficult job (see Chapter 5).

Every aspect of institutionalisation can be seen to have some of its roots in organisational defences against the task. Organisation can, and always does, help and hinder.

Those whose job it is to design, implement and maintain helpful organisation are most clearly, individually and collectively, implicated in constructing anti-task practice and policy, and then requiring the workforce to collude with them. (Front-line workers also initiate anti-task practice and in turn ask managers, unions and policy makers to collude.)

Further hindering organisation takes place (Figure 6.4) as the residential establishment simply becomes an outpost of the bureaucracy which runs it. It relinquishes any direct involvement and responsibility for recruiting and selecting staff; it has no control over who comes in and out of the building; its furniture, equipment and maintenance are within the province of sections of the larger organisation. Decisions about who comes to live there are taken by an admissions panel or section. Officials walk in and out of the building at will and take decisions without reference to residents or staff. Staffing disputes (often about who does what) are negotiated by unions and management outside the building and instructions are issued following an agreement, or a disagreement.

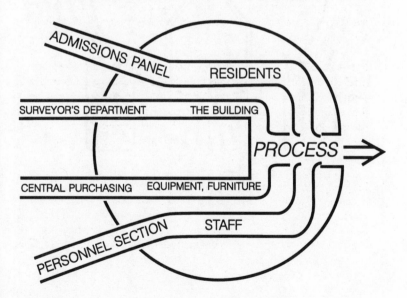

Figure 6.4 A residential establishment as an outpost of a bureaucratic organisation

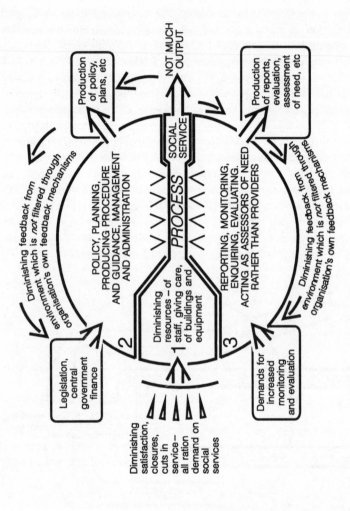

Figure 6.5 A large organisation as three defensive systems

Residents subjected to this process will feel even more estranged from any human and personal contact. In such a situation (which is very common in local authorities and large voluntary organisations) 'relationship work' and the sort of commitment and involvement from staff I have proposed throughout this book will appear to be irrelevant and strange. Such personal work will either be sneered at or rejected as hopelessly old fashioned and impracticable. Staff will cry out for yet more directives and outside guidance, but will reject it when given. Workers, unions and management (and government) will be locked into a pass-the-parcel game with their responsibilities. The primary task will still appear in policy statements; indeed, the rationale for this sort of defensive organisation is often that it is required in order to perform the primary task more effectively. We can see this in bureaucratic responses to new legislation like the Children Act (HMSO 1989).

All new legislation, guidance and management, unless actively reducing laws, rules and procedure, will have a tendency to create defensive systems.

I am not proposing that there should henceforth be no new legislation, nor that we give up on policy development and its implementation. Nor am I implacably opposed to the practical organisation of teams and their work; clearly, in Chapter 5, I am recommending helpful organisation. But it is through our awareness, knowledge and analysis of our management practice that we will resist the hindering aspects of organisation which prevent our application to the primary task. Knowing the potential in organisations for constructing defensive systems, we will be more able to identify those aspects of organisation which distance and divert us from the job in hand.

I have shown by my example of the kitchen cupboard jobs rota how these defences operate within a home. But such seemingly small examples are part of a massive defensive system which is a barrier to good practice in whole organisations even at a national government level. We can see politicians and managers in very senior and influential positions who appear to be oblivious to the process of which they are part.

In Figure 6.5 I illustrate how a larger organisation (for example, a local authority social services department) can also split its functions and focus to defend against the anxiety provoked by the primary task. Central government policy has hastened and colluded with this inherent tendency. By introducing legislation in the health and social services to divide the functions of organisations into 'purchasers' and 'providers', by demanding a constant stream of information and monitoring and by elevating the planning, contracting and bidding process to the highest form of managerial ritual, government has diverted the energy of social service organisations away from *service.*

Figure 6.5 shows three systems at work: system 1, the provision of social service is increasingly squeezed but separated from the other two systems. For a person in need – a user – it is increasingly difficult to obtain a service. It is quite likely that when you ask for a service you will get an assessment of need (system 3) which is then fed back into the planning (system 2) and monitoring process. You are increasingly unlikely to obtain a service unless the organisation has available resources to have contracted with an independent (private or voluntary) organisation to provide the service you require.

Although it is clear that the government has been successfully moving services out of local authority control and into private and voluntary control, I do not suspect that the *intention* has been to reduce the resources given to providing a service and increase the resources given to the attendant managerial and administrative bureaucracy. Indeed, it has long been government's claim that it will reduce such wastage. But this has not been the effect.

The importance of making this point here is to demonstrate the power of unconscious defensive systems when organisations face unmet and anxiety-provoking need. They always respond by creating a well justified, collusive defence. Our struggle in organising residential work will be to identify this process and to resist it even when, as it always will be, it is entrenched in the larger organisations which we deal with or are part of.

THE ROLE OF THE MANAGER

Every small step up the management ladder leads workers away from the primary task and towards secondary tasks. All management and administrative tasks in social services have validity only in their demonstrable aid to the furtherance of the primary task. Given the frightening and anxiety-provoking nature of the primary task and the unconscious organisational tendency to construct defence systems, all managers will find themselves at some point colluding with and even leading this anti-task effort. It is common to hear team leaders and managers in homes pleading the pressures of various forms of paperwork which prevent them from doing the work they profess they would like to do. The massive output of paper and words, usually incomprehensible to non-professionals, serves as a physical and emotional barrier to what is actually happening. The seriousness of response to something going badly wrong (illustrated in Example 6.2) is often measured by how much paper is produced with which to 'wrap it up'; if one report will not do, another is called for and sometimes even a third.

Managers unconsciously collude with this drift away from the task; the more senior the job becomes the more the drift turns into a whirlwind, dragging them into a level of operation which can eventually become completely disconnected from the users of the service (for whom the service exists) and the problems they bring. In the last few years it has become increasingly common for heads of residential establishments and even other senior staff to work conventional office hours.

In my last residential job I spent a lot of energy in my self-management task, attempting to counter the pull of managerialism and to stay with the primary task. I programmed time with residents and with staff, ate with residents, regularly worked parts of shifts with care staff, continued to do on-call duties and usually made time to talk with anyone who asked me for time. This was a major conscious effort and I suggest something similar is required of all managers at every level. I could not meet all the demands of my colleagues and residents in the home, or of my colleagues and managers in the central offices of the organisation (see Chapter 4, Supermanager fantasy, p. 80). Being head of a residential care centre is to be pulled in many directions (Burton 1988), to live with the stress and to direct all your activities to the primary task. This is likely to mean that you will at some time in the week do a bit of nearly all the jobs in the home, meet and talk with nearly all the residents and all the staff; but you will spend a large proportion of your time on boundary issues, at the interface between the residential centre and its environment – the outside world and the wider organisation. All that time and effort spent in meetings, on the phone and writing reports must be directed towards a furthering of the primary task.

The constant and increasing disconnection between management and the primary task is one of the principal causes of breakdown in social service organisations. Every manager who no longer at some time experiences the anxiety provoked by contact with clients or has effectively distanced him or herself from it, has become incapable of managing the task. When bad practice is exposed, basic-grade staff will be categorised as lazy, incompetent, uncaring and unintelligent, and the disconnected manager will invent a new procedure to ensure compliance with the standards she or he has laid down. Failure to meet those standards then results in disciplinary procedures being invoked. Meanwhile, what happens to the resident?

The lure of management and administrative work is strong; the threat of the primary task is even stronger. You will inevitably be simultaneously pulled away from it and repelled by it, and one of your destinations is the Grand Policy Roundabout – a defensive diversion for tired, exhausted and anxious managers and a magnet for the simply ambitious manager. And one of the horses you will ride on the roundabout is Inventing Procedure.

THE POLICY ROUNDABOUT

In my analysis of large organisations I have attempted to interpret their addiction to the production and consumption of policy. (I showed in Chapter 5, Smoking, p. 117 how a children's home, in a parallel process, can become fruitlessly obsessed with control and punishment.)

Dressing up, carrying huge wads of paper, looking particularly serious and sitting for hours in committees with a few dozen others doing the same, is vastly preferable, better paid and of infinitely higher status than assisting a resident with bathing. Yet it is this activity (bathing) which these grave councillors and senior managers are discussing and inventing new procedures for. It is likely that they have not yet asked the resident or the care assistant for their own views, nor are many of them likely ever to have direct experience of this difficult and delicate task (part of the primary task).

In local authorities, elected members (councillors) are responsible for making policy; they do so (usually) in response to new legislation or to adverse reports on their services and on the advice of senior managers, whose job it is to implement policy. This hierarchy of notional responsibilities is similar in most of the larger social service organisations – for instance, the roles of the management committee and senior managers in a voluntary organisation.

Example 6.2   Organisational response to scandal

The daughter of a resident of an old people's home notices bruises on her mother's arms. She has been worried for some time that her mother is not being well treated at the home but her mother is not able to tell her what is going on. The old woman appears to be unhappy, is often dressed in clothes which are not her own and clings to her daughter when she visits.

The daughter has tried to ask the staff about what is going on, but only gets complaints of how difficult the mother is, how she cries and scratches them when they try to dress her or bath her. (One care assistant shows the daughter the scratches on her hands and arms.) They tell her she is incontinent most of the time and has to wear pads (be 'padded up' they say). The daughter knows her mother is difficult to look after; she cared for her

---

for many years before she came to the home where she hoped (and was told) she would get 'professional' care.

After getting nowhere with the care staff, the daughter asked to see the officer in charge. It was two weeks before she was able to see her and when she did she got no further with her enquiries about her mother's welfare. She said she wished to make a complaint and was handed a form to use for that purpose.

News of the complaint circulated in the home and staff were even more reluctant to be the ones to attend to the resident for fear of something else going wrong and triggering another complaint. Some staff felt their jobs were more at risk from doing the job with insufficient resources and support than from not doing it.

The daughter sent the form to the social services headquarters and she got a card saying that her complaint had been received and was being looked into.

In the meantime, her mother had a fall while she was using the lavatory; she was sent to hospital with a broken hip and died of pneumonia a week later.

At about the same time someone from the local authority inspection team had visited the home in response to the complaint, and had discovered in the course of a brief inspection all sorts of major failures in care which had not been spotted in the earlier routine inspection.

However, even the previous inspection had recommended several important improvements. Amongst its more urgent recommendations was an increase in staffing and in training and supervision for care staff. (Particular training needs were identified as Managing Continence and Working with People Suffering from Dementia). These recommendations were the subject of policy discussions at a senior-manager and member (councillor) level but were unlikely to result in any change in the foreseeable future.

The case of the mother's death went to the coroner's court. It emerged that she had entered hospital in clothing which was dirty and smelling strongly of urine and that there were bruises on her upper arms and wrists. The coroner questioned the care she had been given in the home, why she had fallen and how she had got the bruises. There was a sensational report in local paper headlined 'Pensioner Battered and Bruised in Council Care'. Councillors met and called for a full-scale enquiry.

The daughter is now feeling both angry and guilty. She feels she did not do enough about her concerns. She believes that her mother would not have died and would not have suffered if she had not been put in 'that place'. She talks to the press about her experiences at the home and a further, even more revealing story is published.

The enquiry team begins work. They do not expect to report for six weeks. That turns into three months, during which time several other horror stories emerge about this home and others in the same local authority. The council refuses to talk to the press and forbids its staff to say a word about anything that is happening in the social services department.

The enquiry team launches its findings which highlight many longstanding deficiencies in the running of the home, including: under-staffing; lack of training and supervision; divisions and conflict between staff; racism; and a long history of complaints from residents, relatives, staff, social workers and health service staff which had never been properly dealt with. The enquiry team even manage to dig up a report made seven years previously which outlined exactly the same faults.

It is nearly six months since the daughter first expressed her concerns about the care of her mother. Nothing has yet been done to improve the situation in the home. All enquiries have been turned away; some residents have been moved to other homes and some taken away and accommodated by relatives or sent to private homes. Some staff have been suspended pending the outcome of the enquiry and possible disciplinary action.

The home is now staffed by a majority of outsiders, either from other homes in the borough (which were no less short staffed) or from agencies. The standard of care is still much the same as it was but no risks are taken with any residents. Two staff attend to residents at all times. Staff are not allowed to bath residents or take them to the toilet on their own; they must always be accompanied by a colleague, which means in effect that residents get half the attention they previously got. Reports are written on everything that happens and are countersigned by managers. Morale is even lower than it was and no-one wants to work there.

Senior managers respond to the enquiry report by proposing a new use for the home – making it into a 'resource centre' – and forming a working party to produce the new and definitive Procedure Manual which will tell staff at all levels exactly what to do in all circumstances. Four years after the enquiry they are still talking about converting the home to a resource centre or selling it to a private consortium, and the procedure manual (having proved to be no more used than the previous one) gathers dust in the offices of each home.

The policy makers and implementers (councillors and senior managers) do not visit the home and they try to forestall any discussion of it at any public meeting. The inspection unit continues to inspect and report, mostly on what is planned to happen and why as yet it has not been achieved. These reports serve only to lull councillors and senior managers into a false sense of security and blissful ignorance until the next time the cat gets out of the bag, when they will go through exactly the same charade.

All the homes in this organisation have now been subjected to defensive procedures, the stated aim of which is to prevent anything similar ever happening again, but the covert (and largely unthoughtout) purpose is to protect the upper levels of the organisation when something similar does happen. It is as if the organisation deals with its incontinent parts by providing pads and plastic pants ('padding up') rather than playing a positive role in helping to manage good practice – helping people to become continent.

In some homes which were working comparatively well, the areas of good practice which they had established are undermined by the new procedures. Basic-grade workers are still left doing the same job, with the same shortages of staff and lack of resources, but now everything is reported on with the use of new forms and procedures. If the rule says that two members of staff must be present when someone is being bathed (a response to the bruised arms) then imagine what happens when there are not two workers available, which is often the case. The resident does not get her bath, in which case staff must write a report stating why she could not have her bath. Or she must wait until staffing conditions allow her to have a 'fully supervised' bath. (Quite quickly there will be special 'bath days' allocated when sufficient staff are brought on duty to concentrate on bathing.) Or workers risk their jobs, reputation and future employment doing what they know is right, bathing residents on their own and asking for help from a colleague only when they really need it.

Some homes reintroduce the Bath Book in which they record all baths: time, date, 'refusals', staff, any marks or bruises on the resident's body, etc. Of course, no-one fills in the Bath Book with the name of just one care assistant. The record shows that procedures were complied with.

If something goes wrong, like a fall or accidental bruising of an arm (both of which are possible even with two helpers and, of course, very serious), the worker who admits to 'going it alone' will get little support from her union, her managers or her councillors – the very people whose policies, rules and procedures she has had to ignore.

In all social service organisations there is a tendency to draw staff to the centre and away from the clients and the primary task. We can see this in the gradual increase in numbers of managerial and administrative staff compared with the decrease in people who give a service directly to users. We can see it in the trend of legislation and policy, the 'purchaser/provider' split, the idea of 'care management', the massive increase in numbers of people involved in training, consultancy, planning, inspection, evaluation, research and policy formulation. It is an attractive (and much more lucrative) area. It is an area where you do not have to get your hands dirty and you are much less at risk from the troubles which social service users bring with them.

As an officer in charge it may be flattering and a relief to be asked to join a working party which reports to a committee, which in turn formulates a new policy. It is good to be out of the place, away from the stress and risk. It is undoubtedly easier to talk (or write, as in this book) about helping someone with a bath, or helping someone to become continent again, or to advise on the management and control of unruly children and young people than to do it! Ideally, we help to make and implement policy and at the same time are closely involved with the practical work and are supporting others who are closely involved. But it is very easy to find that so much time and energy are taken up with important meetings and high-level talk that what the work itself is like or really about can be quickly forgotten. (This is why this book could be an uncomfortable read for some of the people involved in the 'secondary' areas of work listed above.)

The draw of the policy roundabout is strong and seductive. As soon as we are well settled into our new and important role we will invite others below us to join us, just as we were invited by those above us. We are drawn into an attractive hierarchy which has the effect of increasingly isolating us from the primary task. The more layers of padding we have between us and the frightening realities of the job, the more comfortable we will be and the less effective in improving practice.

Checklist for resisting hindering organisation

*   Observe and analyse your organisation by:
    starting with the daily workings and interaction of where *you* work and the work *you* do;
    moving out by steps to the boundary of your residential establishment and its dealing with the wider organisation;
    being wary of noticing the defences in the wider organisation before identifying those closer to home – such outwardly focused criticism is likely to obscure (and defend against) an awareness of your own defences.
*   Remember the primary task and use it frequently to test the validity of your ideas and actions. Ask yourself the questions 'How will this improve my/our work for residents?' and 'What would residents think about this?' Then try asking them!
*   Be aware of the seductions of power, status and protection from anxiety. You will find that these come in different guises: power

over people is different from power *with* people; status conferred from above is different from status given by those around you; and defence against anxiety is different from support and help to engage with anxiety.

* Practise saying that you need time to think and to talk things over with colleagues and users. A hasty 'Yes' or 'No' is often the opposite of what you might want to say later. Don't just go along with things: you will find yourself caught, unwittingly, in a collusion.

* Within your own part of the organisation, if you invent a new rule or procedure or form to be filled in, go ahead with it only if you find two others which you can get rid of. Then, if you are doing this yourself, try the idea out with the wider organisation. Do a regular stocktaking of rules, procedures and bits of paper to be filled in, and take drastic action if they are increasing. They are enemies of the primary task.

* When in doubt – as you will often be – go for less bureaucracy, less procedure, less organisation, less rule making and following. This is the very opposite of the natural and defensive response to doubt, which is to go for something more certain. (I think of this like steering into a skid to correct it, rather than trying to steer in the opposite direction.)

* Don't automatically equate defensive responses with bad faith on the part of people in power. (My own tendency is to do this.) Remember the unconscious nature of these defences. You are more likely to succeed in resisting such unhelpful organisation if you understand it, help others to understand it, but do not make it a personal campaign.

Chapter 7

Outside assistance

Residential workers require an unusual degree of self-reliance and motivation. I have constantly referred to the difficulties of working in organisations which are unhelpful, unsympathetic and obstructive. I have made a strong case for following ideals, beliefs and principles, and not relying on very much help from the parts of the organisation which are outside the establishment.

But such an attitude can become counter-productive and can lead to defensive, inward-looking, dangerous isolation. The home or centre can become a law unto itself, particularly if there is a strong and charismatic figure in charge. Investigations of dreadful practice in several areas of residential work have featured just such frightening figures. Moreover, they have often been people who were left alone to carry out their own policies, to dominate residents and staff and to deal with problems in their own way.

These scandals would appear not only to justify but to require close supervision and frequent intervention by the managing authorities. But how can we achieve a balance between neglect and interference? How can residential workers use the great potential assistance of outsiders, and how can outsiders develop ways of working which support, guide *and* monitor the residential task without trampling on it?

There who have read from the beginning of this book may, I hope, be saying to themselves, 'The answer's here: the outside process of management, supervision, support and leadership should exactly parallel the inside process.'

I have been moving steadily in my illustrations and discussion towards this point. We started with examining the minutiae, the small, exact details of the work and the focus has been widened, chapter by chapter, until we now come to the point of moving beyond the boundary of the establishment or home to consider the work of the 'outsider'. This does not call for a change of principles or practice because, if we think again for a moment in 'systems', all of the work is in some senses done by outsiders. When Viola and I were working with Mrs Pollard (Chapter 1, pp. 4–6), we were moving in and out of her system – the little area of her bed and its immediate surroundings, her life ebbing away, her dying flesh, her pain and isolation. As we moved across that boundary of her temporary system we created a system ourselves – our work together for twenty minutes with Mrs Pollard. What we then needed was someone outside that system (but within the establishment) with whom we could discuss and reflect on our work: a supervisor. Every other situation described in the book – cooking the tea, the new member of staff, becoming a manager – and every group of staff, every home, can be regarded as a system with a boundary, connecting with people and other systems beyond the boundary. Now we have come to the boundary of the establishment itself and the role of those staff outside who are connected and concerned but are not part of the residential home.

WHAT IS AN OUTSIDER?

Those who neither live in nor regard the establishment as their main place of work are outsiders. A person who visits the home regularly to do some work there – like a psychologist, physiotherapist, chiropodist or central management officer – is usually an outsider. The outsider has a special status and a different potential for helping which the insider does not have. The outsider can quickly lose this useful status by becoming entangled and embroiled and too close, too identified with the inside events, relationships and concerns of the establishment. Equally, outsiders lose efficacy when they, ignorant of the dynamics of residential life and work, circumvent and fail to connect with those inside.

The different sorts of outsider

1 The designated ('line') manager from outside.
2 The people coming in to do a specific job:
   a) social workers, etc;
   b) tutors;
   c) nurses, doctors, pharmacists, etc;
   d) outside consultants – divided into various types:
        i   non-managerial supervision;
        ii group supervision;
        iii group consultant – to special groups;

    iv staff group consultant – staff support/development groups;

    v   organisational consultant;

    vi training consultant;

    vii therapeutic consultant.

3 The inspector.

4 Other official visitors, like councillors or management committee members.

In this brief chapter I will discuss some aspects of the work of only three specific outside roles – those of the line manager, the consultant and the inspector. By doing so I hope to illuminate the work and approach of the others. But first we will look at the cross-boundary interactions and relationships between any outsider and a residential establishment.

Crossing the boundary

Any outsider in a position to manage or help the staff of a residential home with their work, or even working with a client who lives in a residential establishment, and those whose job or duty it is to visit the home needs to know about and to understand much of what has been written about in previous chapters. Residential workers who seek the help of outsiders also need to know in what capacity they want them to work and of what help they may be.

To visit or even phone a residential home from outside is to cross the boundary of a complex and often unpredictable social system. We would expect social workers visiting families to be sufficiently well trained and experienced not to bring with them a set of assumptions about who the family are and how they operate. We would expect them to tread carefully, not to barge in, to observe and pick up the nuances of family interaction but not to jump to conclusions. We need to come into such situations with a full head (knowledge and experience) and an open mind (ready to see and understand things anew). I would expect the same expertise and self-discipline from any professional visitor to a residential establishment. I am often disappointed.

It is unlikely that any visitor will feel at ease, particularly during early visits, in such a complex and charged social setting. Residential homes exist to meet the pressing and sometimes dramatic needs of residents. If I visited an establishment where my needs as a visitor clearly took precedence over needs of residents, or where the needs of residents were not in evidence, I would question its application to the primary task (Chapter 6). However, I might be tempted to collude with this attention

to my needs because it would be more comfortable to do so. An environment which is not orientated to meeting residents' needs will not make
the same challenges and demands on me as one which puts them at the
top of its list of priorities.

(I am already drawing attention to information which you pick up as
an outsider – in any capacity – which will be useful to you and to staff in
the work you do with the establishment, the staff or the residents. You
will pick up information most accurately and quickly by noticing your
own feelings and responses. This information is not available to insiders
unless you give it to them. They don't know what it is like now to be a
visitor to the home in which they live or work, and even if they remember
what it was like when *they* first visited, they were there for a different
purpose – as a potential *insider*. One of the most immediate and direct
examples of differences in insider and outsider perception is the way
people smell a place. The insider soon cannot smell urine if the odour is
permanent; outsiders can, but they usually don't say so. When the outsider
stops noticing the smell, she or he has lost the capacity to contribute to
the development of the home.)

Regrettably, many outsiders still expect the establishment to fit them
rather than for them to find a way of entering, of crossing the boundary
which respects and values the life and work of the place. In Chapter 1, in
the section Local Politics, p. 19 (the committee's visit), instead of enquir-
ing how residents and staff could most conveniently accommodate the
visiting group of councillors these outsiders expected the home to adapt
to *their* needs and, irrespective of all the other urgent needs of residents,
to drop everything and attend to them. Similarly, in the same chapter, I
describe how an assistant director engages in a very important phone call
with which he jeopardises the complex and difficult work being done one
evening in a children's home. These are examples of outsiders' failures
to comprehend the nature of the residential task and the life of residential
homes.

Example 7.1   Visitors not admitted

When discussing how outsiders come in to any residential home, I am
always reminded of an incident at Frogmore (children's home) at a time
when we were straining to contain and hold several children who were 'all
over the place', wild, out of their own control and ours, and very frightened.
As I have described in previous examples, at that time we (the staff) were
trying to provide a calm and well organised setting which had the capacity
to contain and hold such children, and in which we could then engage in

therapeutic work with them. After a particularly harassing and unsuccessful morning, which had involved staff literally holding on to children who would otherwise have climbed on to the roof or run into the street, I was aghast to see two men in suits, carrying clipboards and briefcases, taking photographs and making notes, standing in the back garden. They were council officials working on the fine details of the plans for the alterations which we were having done. In their view they were visiting a council property and were going about their legitimate business. They had no reason to suppose that it was necessary to make an appointment or that they could not just walk in.

My rage was terrible – murderous. My approach to them was hardly less furious. They left quickly having been subjected to a massive discharge from my store of sublimated anger – I 'blew up'! To a detached onlooker it may well have been a farcical scene; to me it was deeply threatening and hurtful, not least to feel such rage against these two, as they thought, innocent parties. They, I suppose, simply thought they had encountered a madman – which in some senses they had! I got some relief and calm only when I had talked with my supervisor, an outsider who understood and helped me to understand.

When we glibly assume that all residential establishments should be open to outside because we are naturally keen on openness and accessibility, we forget the intensely private and sensitive events, the naked and raw emotions, the pain and suffering which are sometimes exposed to view. In one of the most powerful and memorable short passages of writing about residential work, Winnicott (1978, p.152) describes the homes where 'children lie about on the floor, cannot get up, refuse to eat, mess their pants, steal whenever they feel a loving impulse, torture cats, kill mice and bury them so as to have a cemetery where they can go and cry....' In such homes, says Winnicott, there should be a notice: VISITORS NOT ADMITTED.

THE ROLES OF OUTSIDERS

The inspector: scheduled and unannounced visits

Some outsiders who should know about the dynamics of residential life have a role which they believe requires them to turn up unexpectedly, to do spot checks and to ignore the barriers which may prevent their examination of 'what's really going on'. The new arms-length inspectors and registration officers are required to make at least one visit a year without giving notice of their intention to do so. It used to be a common practice of central management officers to call in to residential homes, sometimes, coinciding with a personal visit to shops nearby, or for a cup of tea or coffee on their way to or from work. (See Chapter 2, Example 2.2, A residential management group p. 35.) A very senior manager was once surprised to be told by me that her being an hour late for an appointment meant that those who were to meet with her (me included) were now doing other equally important things and she would have to make another appointment with us. It is still common for social services officers to arrive at a residential home expecting to visit a resident (on business) without making an appointment with the person concerned. This demonstrates a disrespect for the resident and a disgraceful assumption that her or his only role is to be the passive recipient of occasional and haphazard professional attention. A similar attitude spills over towards staff.

The stereotypical view of residential care is powerful and homes with many different styles of life and work are fitted into a convenient and condescending perception. While many outsiders are calling for more participation and activity in residential homes, they can display an under-lying assumption that everywhere staff and residents live a routine and insignificant existence relieved only by the stimulation of contact with busy and benevolent visitors.

They are wrong. As an outsider, coming to a residential establishment on business, you will need to be disciplined and above all courteous. Remember that it is not 'your place' and the people who live and work there have important lives and business of their own to accomplish; you are but one small part of their day.

Of course, there are rare occasions when you *will* need to call unexpectedly. (I am not including social contact between residents and their families and friends, which is their business to arrange how they like.) Usually, on these rare occasions, you will see no more or less than you could have seen on a planned visit, had you known how to look, see, listen, hear, smell and atune to the atmosphere. (See Appendix 3 and Burton 1991b). But you may be worried about something you could not get to the bottom of when they *were* expecting you.

Example 7.2   Picking up clues and taking action

You (a local authority inspector visiting a privately run home) picked up from conversations with the staff and residents that there were some evenings when there were insufficient staff to do the job. When asked, the manager 'proves' to you that there are always three care workers on duty in the evenings; this is corroborated by the rota and other records. You are still not satisfied; the doubts have been sown in different, subtle ways, not least by your overhearing a resident say, 'Aren't we lucky, we've got three of you girls on tonight.' You telephone the manager the next week and say you are still concerned about staffing levels; you tell her why you are concerned and you ask how many staff are on duty that evening. Although the reply is adequate you tell the manager that you intend to call in sometime in the next few weeks to ascertain that sufficient staffing levels are being maintained. Your aim is to ensure that this home is providing proper care. You have picked up (in your planned visit) that in one very important respect this may not be the case and it is your job now to do whatever you can to persuade the management to bring the home up to standard.

The main point I am making about scheduled and unannounced visits is that you should be able to make a comprehensive evaluation during your planned visits (there will nearly always be indicators of bad practice, often in the ways attempts have been made to cover them up) and that unplanned visits should be to follow up, reinforce and pinpoint your recommendations and concerns of the previous visit.

If we take this method of operation back to management practice inside the establishment, we can see how an atmosphere of distrust can sour a whole community. The officers in charge who creep around trying to catch staff out are not doing their jobs properly (Burton 1990a). They should know what is going on without spying on people. However, if this practice is set up by outsiders it becomes endemic, and weak managers follow a destructive lead encouraging staff simply to 'watch their backs' and not to get caught out.

The management officer

(Throughout the following discussion I refer to heads of homes or officers in charge as if they alone make decisions and take responsibility for the whole home. it will be clear from the previous chapters that I do not recommend such an autocratic style of management. I use the terms for the sake of simplicity and brevity to represent the management of the home however it is organised.)

In the early 1970s, when social services departments were new, the outside manager was called the 'homes adviser'. Later, 'manager' was more common as part of the title – group manager, service manager, homes manager. It has always been a difficult and ill-defined job, and people doing it have often found themselves caught between their commitment to and, for some, direct experience of working in residential care, and their commitment to the organisation (department).

In practice, the creation of a new level of management outside residential centres has frequently confused issues of responsibility and discretion. When it was once clear that the manager (the head, the officer in charge) had the job of managing the home *and* its dealings with the outside world, with the advent of homes advisers it was often quite unclear who had what responsibilities in relation to the management of an establishment. And, in most organisations, it remains unclear. In large bureaucracies, as we have seen in Chapter 6, it is quite possible for several central managers – and even trade union officials or environmental health officers – all to believe they manage separate aspects of a home's functioning. This multiplicity of management results in an unintegrated service.

The formal organisation does, of course, have a profound influence on the management of residential homes but it does not have to dictate the whole way people do their jobs. Workers in homes do need supervision, support, consultation and expert advice, plus a designated line manager who has responsibility for a group or section of the residential service *and* who, most significantly, can take decisions which relate to the *group or section* for which she is responsible. This is what we were requiring of the head of home but with a wider spread of responsibility. It *is* difficult to accomplish the tasks of supervision, support, consultation, advice and line management responsibilities in one role, but we expect the same spectrum of tasks of every manager wherever they are in the organisation and however wide their span of responsibility is spread. But overlapping and duplication of areas of responsibility and discretion create areas of conflict and make for poor management and a poor service.

It is here that the ideas of a boundary and inside and outside are especially useful. The head of home is responsible for what goes on in the home (applying resources of people, place and plant to the primary task) and for those transactions which take place across the home's boundary. Similarly, the group manager is responsible for managing the primary task of a group of homes and the transactions across the boundary of her section or group. They are responsible for different levels of the service. In a similar way, the head of home has assistant managers who are responsible for specific areas of the home's functioning, like a group living unit or training and development or catering.

The notion of boundary is essential to performing helpful outsider roles. The group manager's job is to help, support, advise, counsel, guide and consult with the head of home but *never* to cross the boundary and manage the home. The relationship between the two managers will at times be difficult and precarious, especially when they are engaged with an issue on the boundary between their two roles.

There always comes the point when the manager of a home is being asked to take residents which she does not believe she should take. (See Chapter 1, p. 18) This decision is the head of home's. When the head of home says 'No' and the department or wider organisation is saying 'Yes', the temptation for the outside manager (often under extreme pressure from those above her) is to take the decision away from the head of home. This is often the start of withdrawal away from responsibility by both the head of home and the outside manager. The boundaries of responsibility have been broken and are difficult to replace. In no time at all decisions about admissions climb further up or are dispersed within the organisation. The head of home has lost a crucial element of her boundary responsibilities and loses authority and the capacity to manage effectively.

Leaving the responsibility (the exercise of discretion) with the head of home does not of course mean that whatever she says goes and there is nothing anyone can do about it. She has been selected for the job on the basis that she can and will take that responsibility and use her discretion wisely and well. If she does not, this is exactly the sort of area in which the outside manager will be exercising her responsibility to provide supervision. In supervision the head of home will be 'Held, listened to, encouraged; Challenged, confronted, stimulated; Disciplined, informed, answerable' (Houston 1990). But she still has to take the responsibility for making a decision that is part of *her* job.

Clarity about boundaries of the respective roles and a sharp awareness of insider/outsider status and relationship are the basis of a productive working partnership between the head of home and the line manager.

The outside consultant

I have practised as an outside consultant in all the various ways I have listed under 2(d) on pp. 145–6. In two periods of freelance work, 1979–82 and 1987 to the time of writing, I have been involved with many different organisations, groups and individuals. I have used a variety of training and educational courses, constant reading and supervised practice to develop my work. Yet I still find myself stymied and floundering.

Involvement as an outsider is hard, especially for someone, like me, who has been an insider and identifies strongly with insider concerns. I have taken care to be honest in this book about where I stand, about my views and beliefs. This process of writing is itself an outsider activity: I am an outsider to you, the readers and your places of work. I try to blend the authentic me, my experience, my thoughts and feelings in ways which you can use. I have tried to avoid overloading the book with instruction and advice, without artificially holding back information which I think will be of use; to offer ways of thinking about things and reflections on real practice issues which you can use – directly, now; not to be dogmatic about the way you go about your work but to have it in mind as I write.

Different readers will receive this in different ways. Some may find my use of examples and personal reflection (like now) overdone and too specific to mean anything in *your* situation; and others will find that knowing about me in my work helps them to know about themselves in their work. I run many risks by not staying on the well-trodden path of producing a book full of other writers' thoughts and theories, examples of other people's practice and adaptations of other authors' guidelines and procedures.

My experience as a training consultant is that the encouragement to become personal is rejected by many groups. The groups more likely to use and learn from their own experience – both current experience at work and during a course – are groups of care assistants, home helps and basic-grade workers in any area of residential care. They are usually willing and able to join in a cooperative learning endeavour (see Appendix 1, Learning Basket) which the trainer or consultant helps to get started by being personal and vulnerable. To some other groups, usually those with more training and in higher-status jobs, this is an embarrassing challenge which is dismissed as 'not teaching us anything' or 'didn't seem to know what he was talking about'.

Surely, the more training a worker has received and the more sophisticated his work the more we might expect him to have developed the capacity to learn from experience. But previous training and current supervision (if it has existed) may have served only to increase his detachment from and his defences against the pain and anxiety of the job. Experiential learning, unless completely separated from work, will only rekindle the discomforts experienced before erecting the defences and may therefore itself be rubbished and dismissed.

Often, when working as a training consultant, I find there is no channel through which to feed this information back into the organisation, and attempts to create that channel are blocked. The staff are acting out the defences of the organisation which responds to the training in the same way, calling it 'inappropriate' (a favourite word) and too basic, with not enough information and guidelines and the trainer being not 'expert' enough.

Of course, when I get this sort of feedback I become as defensive and insecure as the people I describe above! I rely on supervision to help me to distinguish between what *I* need to work on to improve *my* performance and what I should feed back to the organisation I am working for. Complimentary feedback is also worth analysing and not merely basking in!

The satisfactions and frustrations of training are present in all other forms of consultancy. Acting as a consultant to a staff team to help them to develop and maintain effective working relationships and to share their concerns and anxieties is taxing work. Having been a residential worker, I have a strong empathy with those I am working with: I understand their frailty and difficulties. I therefore have to work hard at staying in my outsider role. Early in my consultancy experience I found that I was over-compensating by distancing myself, and although I was using my own feelings and experience to understand and interpret what groups brought to meetings, I never revealed them. As my confidence grew I relaxed more and accepted that I too could make mistakes, and that sometimes my mistakes could free people in the group to take risks and make their own mistakes. A proper balance is rarely achieved by staying still in precisely the right place; it is more likely that we keep moving to one side or the other of the point of balance.

Very few residential establishments use, or are afforded the resources to use, outside consultancy. In my various residential management jobs I have had only occasional access to independent consultants, but I have sometimes been given good supervision within the organisation and have found some training courses gave me opportunities for high-quality consultation.

The outside consultant is often asked into an organisation to do something about a problem or group of staff. Adults seeking autographs from celebrities often say, 'It's for my niece' (or nephew or someone similar), and it can be like that with a first approach about consultation. A manager will phone about a group of staff she or he manages: '*They* need some training' or '*They* need some team-building' – a current favourite. '*They*' are usually people in the organisation who are lower in the hierarchy than the person asking for the help. It is quite likely that the manager has tried all sorts of ruses to improve the performance of the group of staff he has in mind; he turns to consultation as a last resort.

When I am faced with this situation I ask a lot of questions. I expect any request for consultancy to have several levels of meaning and history.

I start working with the enquirer as soon as we speak. I want to know what has led up to the request; what is the presenting problem and what is the history of dealing with this problem. I ask what prompted this phone call – has something happened or has pressure been put on the caller and by whom?

If we arrange to meet for the next stage of consultation I usually make it clear that I start charging at this point. This helps people to do some work on the issue beforehand and improves the chances of a purposeful meeting. I will often write to them after we have met to sketch out what I thought the issues were and how I think I may be able to help, if I think I can.

I learned this way of operating from taking referrals for new residents. The process is essentially the same. You need to know as much as you can about the context of the referral, what the referrer has done and what they are expecting you to do. You need to ascertain whether this is, in the view of the referrer, more a positive choice or a last resort. You need to know what the person (or team) being referred thinks about it – are you expected to do something *to* them or are they keen to start work *with* you? You need to meet to begin a process of assessing and planning.

Whether it is a new resident or a team engaging with outside consultation, in most instances the work stands little chance of success if the process is imposed. Nearly all successful consultative work is based on an equal partnership between the parties. I will not enter into work with a team unless they have made a decision to engage me. I meet with them; we weigh each other up; we explore and decide on the way we wish to work. We negotiate our agreement, which always includes reviewing the process and leaves either side the power to end the agreement. In other words, they hire and fire me. I write to the team as a group and I usually send my bill to them; I think it is helpful for them to know *all* the terms on which they have engaged me.

Sometimes I work with several levels in an organisation, but I have to be careful to spell out the boundaries of confidentiality and to make sure all the groups and individuals I am working with know that I am working with the others. Secret meetings with secret agendas destroy confidence in the consultant and undermine confidentiality.

Again, the principles and practice I am advocating here I learned in residential work. By using them as a consultant to residential workers I am helping to maintain them in practice with residents. I am acutely aware that my behaviour, attitudes and ways of working as an outsider are often as influential as the work I have been hired to do. Again, the parallel with being a residential worker is exact.

All of us who work in residential care know how much help we can obtain from outside, but we also know how hindering and clumsy outsiders can be. I have two friends (one is my current supervision partner) in whose houses shoes are not worn. For me, there is something in the act of taking off my shoes at the front door which reminds me of the way I like to go into a residential home as an outsider: I have accepted the ways of the house and its residents. I know that these ways signify important aspects of religion, culture and philosophy. I make a small but significant act of acknowledgement and I do not feel weaker, or less equal, or put down by doing so. In a residential home I wish to make clear that I am sensitive and knowledgeable about what is or may be going on, that I know life and work in this place is complicated and often difficult, that things are not always what they appear to be, and yet I retain my independence, my perception and my own principles. I go in carefully, considerately and critically. And I leave with insights and very personal information about other people which I will keep safely and work on for *their* benefit, not for mine nor for that of prying bystanders.

Chapter 8

A good place to live?

This chapter is the result of a series of interviews with people who are or have been residents, which I conducted towards the end of writing this book. Constraints of space have meant that I have had to select just four stories. Three are from people I have worked with who are now friends, two of them close friends. I do not claim that these four accounts of residential care represent what the majority of users would say if several hundred interviews were to be conducted in a major survey; that I do not know. But I *am* sure that they identify many of the issues which concern other residents I have heard from over the years. Nor do I discount the affects of my personal and (earlier) professional connection with my three friends, although they do not spare their criticisms of the care homes and social services in which I worked.

The purpose of the chapter is to introduce some direct comment on residential care from those for whom it exists. Each account will repay very close scrutiny; there is a wealth of vital information for care workers, managers and policy makers. Nearly every sentence makes a clear point from which lessons can be drawn on improving residential care.

I have not revised other chapters in the light of these interviews but a good deal of my approach to residential work has been directly influenced by listening to users, and there is considerable support here for a lot of what I have tried to say in the other chapters. (Note: it was necessary to disguise the identity of some of the people in these accounts and therefore, for the sake of consistency, all names of people and places have been changed.)

BOUNDARIES ARE IMPORTANT BUT BROKEN RULES AREN'T THE END OF THE WORLD: JOE'S STORY

Joe came to Chaucer Place after a period of using drugs, prison, a 'de-tox' in Kent and a short period in a local detoxification centre.

A few things happened in my life which swung me in the direction of this place. You can generally tell people who have been in a re-hab; they're weird. At one time I used to try to avoid getting in places like this. I'd heard that Chaucer Place was opening. It was known in the drugs field that a new place was opening on the manor. This is my area. I grew up here. My sister lives a few yards away. The house I grew up in is fifteen minutes walk away. I know everyone.

It was my decision to come. And it was in my area – so it just stuck in my mind. I'd tried it away from my area and it hadn't worked, and in any case no matter where I was to come off drugs, I've still got to come back home.

I knew the first thing I wanted to do when I came out of prison was to take some drugs. But being locked up again was something I wanted to avoid in the future at all costs. The thieving which had provided the money to buy drugs was becoming more difficult because I had to be more careful with the reality of prison hovering over me.

I missed the first appointment I made because I was stoned. I turned up to the next interview an hour late because of a misunderstanding. On the third attempt my sister came with me to make sure I got to the interview. I asked her to give me a bit of support.

I was quite relaxed on the first day. I knew a couple of people and they showed me around. I felt more at home because I knew the area. The building has quite an inviting look to it. Although I didn't feel nervous, people told me later that I really looked nervous.

At the beginning of the programme, it's fairly easy. For the first four weeks you're not allowed out without an escort. The information you get given to start with and the written stuff didn't really sink in. I learned about the place and the programmes as I went along and particularly from other residents who then seemed to look out for each other and help each other. They tell you before the staff tell you, which is a good thing, because if the staff have to do it all the time you get the feeling they're digging you out.

I thought I had it perfectly under control to begin with, but as you go along things begin to pop up. Things surface that have been hidden for so long. They catch you by surprise. I re-established contact with my daughter, getting to know her, visiting her at weekends. I began feeling things after about six weeks.

I was very keen to get involved with everything which was going on to begin with. I was still getting the drugs out of my system and quite often feeling unwell. I was angry about everything but I kept it under control. Sometimes I felt like shit and I'd be told it was my turn for washing up or something like that. It was hard. I spent a lot of time in the kitchen when I first came here; keeping busy kept my mind off how ill I was feeling. I used to take control; basically I like to be in control.

The residents can run the place if they choose to take it on, but if they choose not to then the staff will do everything and then the residents have got the cheek to scream about it. Early on I was very active in participating with the planning and managing of activities, negotiating with staff. We decided we wanted a bit more say about what goes on the menu. I put myself across well. I can make myself understood. The staff encouraged this. I can organise well which I do a lot in my own family too.

We have a meeting every morning to decide what we're going to do and who's going where. And then the staff have a meeting once a week and a resident can go along. I was often the representative who attended the staff meeting.

Being a 'senior resident' is important: the residents who have been here longest should set an example but towards the end of my stay I set a bad example.

The atmosphere is not the same at Chaucer Place now. There was a safe atmosphere but there seems to be a lack of community spirit at the moment. But it is always different looking back.

The staff are here to assist you in what you need, and sometimes to open your eyes a bit to what you need. They suggest things but you decide and then they will help you if you ask. When you're taking diabolical liberties you can rely on them to put their foot down.

Boundaries are really important. The residents have control but if you abuse your power it's taken off you. I need the occasional kick up the arse.

The safety was important. If you felt like crying you could, in front of everyone; it didn't matter. It was nice to know the staff were there. I had a couple of members of staff who I particularly got on with. There was one of these I was frightened of – I couldn't take any liberties with her, but she was always there to support me. She took over a bit of a mum role to me. I cried on her shoulder many a time. My mum died when I was very young. I could rely on her to pull me up sharp before things got too bad; she could recognise when things were going wrong for me.

I knew that I had the affection and respect of this member of staff – even when I was being told off. I felt I was a little bit special to her. Every resident needs to feel that with someone on the staff. The keyworker system didn't really work well for me; I didn't get on with my keyworker but I found a lot of what I needed from other members of staff.

I've been living away from Chaucer Place for three months but I'm in close touch because I use the day centre twice a week and staff are still helpful, and pull me up sometimes – even to the extent of me being suspended.

There is a strict rule in the place that residents may not form sexual relationships with each other. If this happens people are warned off at first but if the relationship continues they will be told to leave or be suspended. The reasoning is that such an exclusive relationship will cut the couple off from the rest of the community and from the work they both need to do for themselves. The couple may be colluding to fight off the effects of what's meant to be happening in the place. I fully agree with the reasoning behind this rule but for reasons of my own I broke the rule and had to take the consequences.

Testing rules is part of learning and growing. Boundaries and rules are essential. Staff have to accept that broken rules aren't the end of the world. I went through some bad times at Chaucer Place as well as good. I gave staff a rough time and was stubborn, devious and sore-headed sometimes, but it was partly through these difficult periods that I learned and staff managed to stick with me. I am a well respected and very involved member of the community. My stay didn't follow an ideal pattern. Near the end I was panicking that I hadn't yet managed to get involved in any voluntary work which is a regular part of most people's programme, and I'm very aware of all the things I didn't learn.

I was very scared about leaving. I didn't know if I could cope but I wanted to try it out.

I attend the day centre twice a week, and sometimes I run the sessions myself. I'm doing a counselling course, and working in a youth club. I value the structure which Chaucer Place has helped me to build, and the support and advice I still get from staff. It's still very difficult sometimes to keep on my chosen path. I'm very short of money. At times the temptations of the old life are strong. But I feel I have a lot to offer now and being at Chaucer Place has helped me to know what I can give.

PACKED OFF AND FORGOTTEN: THERESA'S STORY

I first went to a children's home when I was twelve. I was brought up in Ireland, in the country. When I came to England I lived with my mother and brother. I had a secure childhood in Ireland but things changed for me when I came to England. We had no money and my mother became ill.

I was ahead at school. I had a very good education, a good school report. I loved football.

My mother had a breakdown and we were taken into care. My school contacted the social services.

For my first year in care, I had no social worker.

I can remember arriving. It was June – a sunny day. I played football in the back garden. The people who ran the home were called Aunty Betty and Uncle Paul – that's what we had to call them. The home was by the sea.

I was pleased to get away from my mother – it was a relief. I met Zoë, my best friend. But the school wasn't suitable for me. The head teacher looked at me in a funny way.

Staff at Fairhaven didn't know we bunked off school. Anyway, I wasn't supposed to go to school for the first few months; I went on holiday in Switzerland with the home instead.

The staff left us to our own devices. They didn't take much notice of us but they were strict in a way. We played football but I can't remember much more.

I remember spending summer making camps.

Every Saturday we got our pocket money and walked up to the village. I used to buy the latest football magazine.

I was nervous at school. I couldn't participate. I decided to skive.

I was interested in the social life. We went to a disco every week by bus. Just me and Zoë.

I used to run away a lot. I tried four times. I dreamt of how happy I was – had been. I didn't have a social worker and I had no news of my mother. I wanted to get back to London.

We used to nick things from the shops on Saturdays.

I was at Fairhaven for about a year. School was the source of a lot of the problem and not having a social worker and no contact with home. I was packed off and forgotten.

There were hardly any staff at Fairhaven. It wasn't that I didn't like them. A husband and wife team used to come in and do the cooking and the cleaning. There was nothing like talking with staff on the level like at Northfield.

I nearly drowned. Something happened and I went by the sea and I thought the police were after me.

I wasn't frightened of the staff at Fairhaven but they wore me down. They threatened me with not going to Switzerland again. But I did eventually get away.

I got a train. Tom [social worker] picked me up from Charing Cross. They stopped me for not having a ticket.

The police gave me a cigarette. I was fourteen. But it was the social worker who frightened me. He wouldn't tell me where I was being taken; he said, 'You'll discover that when we get there'. That's what scared me. It always sticks in my mind. The police were alright. The social worker was embarrassed when he met me later.

I was taken to Northfield – by two men. [Social worker and policeman: male nurses are still intruding into young women's rooms in hospital.]

I remember Northfield was sheddy – not looked after – when I first arrived. That was my first impression. I was free at Northfield. Fairhaven was about material comfort. I was glad to be back in London.

My room was important to me. I look back and I had really happy times at Northfield.

I don't think people really appreciated how not going to school affected me. The staff tried to get me to go. I wanted to go but I couldn't. I was too far behind. Zoë takes things in her stride but things worry me.

I remember Ben [staff] a couple of days later introducing himself. That sticks in my mind. And I remember Jill [staff] – I liked her.

It was a comfort seeing young staff. I dreaded one of the cleaners. She bossed people around. The cleaners invaded our private lives. I didn't want the cleaners passing judgement on me. I felt everyone knew my business. They made assumptions about me. They forgot I was from Ireland – I'm not a city girl.

The staff tried to get me to go to school. It was just a short stay – just six or seven months. I wanted to stay. Why was I only able to stay a short time? I was angry at being moved.

I went on to a girls' hostel. But school was a big problem. Then I was only there three or four months then I went to the adolescent unit of a psychiatric hospital. That was bad.

But all this time from fourteen to thirty-three I've stayed in touch with Northfield. I was happy and free. I had contact with my mother. I could choose to see her. My social worker used to come regularly. She never let me down.

It was a happy period for us all [Northfield]. We were all meant to tidy the place up on a Saturday morning and I remember being told that I must sweep the yard before I got my pocket money but Zoë wasn't told that. I used a few words of abuse. I wrote on the board in the kitchen: 'Tim Banbury is a bastard'. We were only joking.

There was a meeting about me when I was breaking up my records. I threatened a boy with a cigarette. He was goading me. There was this special meeting about my behaviour. They were in a little room.

I was forced to go to the meetings. I thought I might not be allowed to stay if I didn't go to the meetings. It was never said. Not like at the therapeutic community I lived in later.

It's your home at the time. You can't keep threatening people with being told to leave. That didn't happen to me at Northfield.

I saw Tim as someone who was stable. The head didn't have much to do with us. He was older and I was used to having older people on my back. There was Tim and Ben, and Pauline that I did have something to do with. I chose to stick to a couple of members of staff. I chose who I wanted to relate to.

At Fairhaven I was in the middle of nowhere.

When I was at Northfield, I used to go to the discos – Young Socialist discos! Zoë and I went. I was told that I had to be back at a certain time and if I was late the door would be shut, but when I did come back late Tim never came down heavy on me. He encouraged me to go to the disco, said it would do me good. I was shy.

I used to keep Ben up. Sitting at the kitchen table smoking. We went for a walk one night. We were standing on Wandsworth Bridge and he was saying how nice the city looked at night. I couldn't see it at the time – it wasn't like the country but I know what he meant now.

If the staff give some of their background to you, it may seem nothing at the time, but in years to come the importance comes through. I remember Terry would say to staff, 'If I don't know anything about you, why should you know anything about me?'

Staff have to give something of themselves.

Children are labelled inferior. The staff can still be staff *and* be personal.

At the hospital adolescent unit it was authoritarian – injections if you didn't behave. Drugs to control you. You don't know how you stepped out of line but you still got drugged. After the girls' hostel and Northfield it was terrible to be locked up. The staff were of the same age but they had a totally different attitude. I was just fifteen.

I cried when I left that unit. I don't know why; I just cried and cried. My social worker was with me. She stuck with me all the time and she kept in contact with my mother while I was at the unit.

I went to the therapeutic community in the country after the hospital. I lost my London connection for a while. But three people from Northfield came to see me there. Over time it was good although some of the staff were bitches. I stayed there for a year and a half – the longest I was anywhere since I came over from Ireland.

I haven't met anywhere in these last ten years when I've been ill like Northfield. Places can go through good and bad times. At Northfield and the therapeutic community there were particularly good staff at the time.

The essential thing is that staff are personal. It's too much of a hassle for children to keep the place nice. Pocket money should be just given – it's yours. Washing-up rotas don't work. There should be people paid to do that.

On the other hand, there are things that children should do. But it shouldn't be organised – it's too much. It's the size of places. To be homely places mustn't be too big.

When I was sixteen they tried to foster me. It didn't work. We had political arguments. I was back with my mother two months later.

IF I'M GOOD THEY'RE GOING TO KEEP ME; IF I'M BAD THEY'RE GOING TO MOVE ME: SANDRA'S STORY

I was in a nursery until I was nine months old but I first went to live in a children's home when I was seven. I had been fostered before but that broke down. I liked the home – it was small and I got attention. It was like a family. I was the youngest. He [the housefather] used to tell me stories every night. He never had a book; he told the stories out of his mind. I remember them and he used to sing songs too. There were children with different needs and disabilities.

When I went there I was speaking French because I'd lived in Paris. But I lost all that. I was only there about a year. Then I went to a reception and assessment centre. It was awful. They weren't very nice to me. It was a big place with loads of children. I don't know what happened to me but I could have been abused there – I don't know. But then I remember everything horrible that I've done and has happened to me. At this place we had to queue for our food and then eat it quickly. But if we put our mouths too close to our plates a woman in a blue suit would come and push your head in your food and everyone laughed at you. It happened to me with rice pudding. I felt like a prisoner.

Later when I went to another home it was much nicer and the food was put out on the tables for you to help yourself. But I'd got used to one system where you had to grab the food to get any, so I did that at this place and I got rapped over the knuckles with a spoon for being greedy.

I was like a little parcel being passed around. In Paris I slept in a room with a little boy who had no legs.

When I look at the places I had to live in... I feel sad. It reminds me of my own daughter and what would be happening to her at the age she is now. I don't think she could cope. She isn't as strong as I am... as I had to be. I was always passed about. That's wrong; you should never do it to a child.

A child thinks, 'If I'm good, they're going to keep me; if I'm bad they're going to move me. Do they really love me or are they just doing a good job?' Later I used to think they've only been nice to me to get a good report out of me for the evening.

Look at me here in this picture [she shows a picture of herself with about a dozen other children] thrown in with all the rest of them.

No love at that reception centre. I only remember that one staff who pushed my head in the pudding.

I then went to another home. It was brilliant; I loved it there. These people brought a massive great teddy bear and sweets. They took my photograph and really made me feel welcome. There was a boy there who I knew from a previous home. It was good to see someone I knew. They moved him on because he was naughty.

I did naughty things to get attention. I was so desperate for attention, love and cuddles. I always thought they were going to move me on – I knew they were going to move me on. I wanted to see if I was naughty would they still keep me. I used to be told that by them. I threw things at staff. I was more violent than any children they had seen. They said they couldn't cope and if I didn't change I was going to have to leave. I said I didn't care if I left because they always moved me around anyway. Really I just wanted them to give me a cuddle and say it's alright, you are going to stay here.

I can remember coming to Northfield. I came with my best friend and Sister Jane. Two boys came to the door and said, 'Yeah, what do you want?' They shut the door in my face. No staff came to welcome me. Everyone was in that horrible dining room – it was awful.

There was a cat. I loved that cat. There were kittens and I killed one accidentally. I was washing it and it got pneumonia.

Although I'm of mixed race, I was brought up – in the various places I'd lived – in a very White society. There were so many Black people at Northfield. It was a shock to me. I was frightened. I don't like saying this; I'm not proud of it but it's the truth. I was the youngest there; it was awful. There were no staff when I needed them.

I remember it all very clearly. Tony wanted to kill me because it was his kitten that died. He used to kick my little legs. I had skinny little legs.

When Tim and Stella were on duty I felt safe. Stella used to do my hair, grease it and plait it. She was all motherly. She used to tell me how pretty I was and what a nice colour my skin was. I used to go to Tim's house with his family at weekends with my friend Camilla. I remember Tim coming and reading stories to me and Camilla at night. Stella never read stories but she used to cook nice dinners – whatever I wanted she used to cook.

Diane [an older girl] was nice to me as well – she used to look after me. And I used to get on Naomi's [another older girl] nerves because I used to follow her around for protection. There was this gang of younger boys (older than me) who made my life hell.

One thing I liked about Northfield (at the beginning) was the clothing allowance. Before I used to have second-hand clothes – things which were given. Pocket money as well – that was good.

You can tell when staff really care about you. I can't explain it. Firm but really good to be with; I really felt secure when I was with Tim. But then when he was on duty I didn't want anyone else to have the attention.

I remember one community meeting – it was after Tim had left. it was when I came back to live at Northfield later – I was older then. I hit a boy in the face and made his nose bleed. I was told if I didn't say sorry to him I would have to leave. They would get the police and I would be done for assault. I really didn't want to say sorry. Sid [one of the staff] said to me quietly, 'Just say sorry, just say sorry. If you do it'll be forgotten about.' I said sorry. I'd been kicked out of my previous home again and come back to Northfield but then I was sent away to a lock-up place.

They thought I was going to get pregnant so I was sent to be locked up. I was going out a lot. They thought I was out of control and two other girls had got pregnant. I was fourteen.

It was all girls at the lock-up place. Funnily enough I liked it because it was secure. We never went out. The staff there were alright. If you swore three times you used to get locked up for twenty-four hours – I didn't like that very much. I grew up a bit when I was in there.

I then got sent back to Northfield again but the new head decided I should go back to the same lock-up place but this time in the secure part of it where you were locked up all the time. I don't know why – it'll be in my files.

It always seemed like I was too naughty for the place I was kicked out of but too good for the places I was sent to.

I didn't mind living in the secure unit – I felt secure. The responsibility had been taken off me. It's not normal but I began to like it. It's not right. The other girls used to say they couldn't wait to get out and I pretended to agree but when I did leave I started to cry. Then I was sent to another secure unit; I liked it there too. I stayed for a year.

Tim came to see me there but I wasn't allowed to see anyone but my social worker. I did my CSEs there – and got good grades. I felt secure there too. We never went out. For one year I stayed in – locked up. I liked it there because we were so close. The staff were always around – it was nice.

I had to be so strong – specially early on when I was little. I'm too strong – hard. I don't even trust people close to me sometimes. But I can give all my love to my daughter – every little bit because I don't feel she's using me. Other relationships are difficult. I can't put all of myself into them; I don't want to be hurt any more. When something goes wrong, I can cry and I'm upset but it goes quickly.

I hate it when I put people down but I can't help it sometimes.

I CHOSE TO COME HERE; I MANAGE WELL: MRS DUNSFORD'S STORY

I have lived here for eleven years. I came straight from hospital which I think was the best way. I had two friends who lived here and I chose to come here because of them. I said to one of them I'd like to come and she said, 'You can't, we're full. There are 119 people here already!' But I did manage to get in. There were crowds of people downstairs; you could hardly get a seat. Some of the residents were in a poor state but it seems like there are even more sick people now. But it's been built up a lot now.

I couldn't go on living at home. Although I had a home help and meals on wheels, and lots of other help, I was still on my own a lot. I had become very disabled – unable to walk. My family are very caring but I was very worried that I was just too much for them, though they never said so. I was lonely too and would stare out of the window all day. I could count the leaves on the trees.

I liked a lot about the old days here. I used to meet different people everyday and I remember all the old staff. I see some of them now. We used to have a jolly good laugh. I remember Moira taking her shoes off to get me into bed. I said, 'I've heard of Sandie Shaw taking her shoes off to sing but I've never heard of taking your shoes off to help someone to bed.'

I liked a lot of the staff especially the ones who helped me. I love to see the ones I used to know then and the domestic workers. But the staff now on my floor are very good.

I like some of the changes – things like the shop and the hoists. The hoist makes life easier for me and for the staff. It's the only thing that really worries me – not being able to use the toilet on my own. But the hoist makes it easier and more dignified. I like staff who treat me with respect – men or women, it doesn't matter, as long as I trust them and they are respectful and business like. Edward was ever so good – he was a proper gentleman.

If staff don't act properly, I can say so. We have a meeting and sort it out, and then it's all forgotten.

As we are now, I think the staff understand one another and work well together. If they don't it affects me badly because I need their help so much.

It's sometimes difficult to get on with other residents. I do my best. I feel mean if I can't say, 'Good morning and how are you?' but sometimes people seem to be completely cut off or are very edgy. One resident who's been here a bit longer even than I have, you have to go a bit easy with her because you can upset her. I can say, 'What a lovely day it is' and she'll say, 'It's cold outside'. I take an interest in all the other residents; I talk to nearly all of them and try to help if I can. I remember when I thought I was losing my mind. When I was at home. I was very frightened and I think I know what it's like if you are seeing things and imagining all sorts of things that aren't really happening – but they're real enough to the person suffering.

I get up early. I could get up later but I can't let myself trouble the day staff. So the night staff bring me a cup of tea and help me to get up. They're very good. Violet brought me a cup of tea this morning. You know what she calls me? – Supergran. She has a family and she's very understanding; I feel at ease with her. Lots of the staff have grown-up children and I remember some of them when they were little.

I do a lot for myself; I manage well. I've got all sorts of little ways of helping myself and I've arranged the room so I can manage. I can wash myself although the basin isn't really in the right place – it's awkward with my wheelchair. Having a TV with remote control means I can lie in bed and watch – sometimes I go off to sleep with it on.

I need staff who let me take things at my own pace. I've worked out ways of doing things. People who know me are wonderful because they know exactly what to do and everything has to be done in the right order. But staff who don't know me aren't much help.

I feel safe here. I've got the bell if I need anything. I don't like being dependent for some things, but I am and that's the fact of the matter. I have to have help and once I've accepted it, then it's easier for me and for the person helping me. I chose to come here.

They used to come up with our pensions but now we go down to collect them. Then I see people I haven't seen for some time which is very nice.

One of the most important things is keeping the toilets clean. I don't have any worries about saying to a visitor that they can go and use the toilet – I know it'll be alright. People are bound to make a little mistake sometimes but the important thing is to *keep* them clean.

Chapter 9

Liberating institutions
A future for residential care

PAST, PRESENT AND FUTURE

At a time of potential for major change in residential care we seem to be stuck, frightened and frozen, apparently more concerned with stopping things happening than enabling them to happen. We know of the conscious and unconscious forces ranged against making positive changes. We have analysed the performance of organisations when engaged with people's deep and urgent needs, and we know there will always be a tendency to eliminate risk and minimize pain and anxiety. However, current legislation and public policy provide opportunities for bold changes with which we could make a reality of 'positive choice' in residential care (NISW/HMSO 1988, *The Wagner Report*).

In this chapter I describe in some detail part of a vision I have for the future – community care centres – and I discuss ways of achieving change. This book has not provided a neat set of theories and instructions of how to assemble the finished article. Similarly, in this chapter, my vision of one part of the future is not a blueprint. It is an idea to be adapted and added to, to be discussed and to lead to other ideas. It is based on many other people's ideas and experience.

Most of my own experience as a residential worker *is* positive. There is much that is positive in the varied experiences and ideas of the residents and ex-residents who tell their stories in Chapter 8. I do not pretend that residential care is universally good; we all know that much of it, in all its forms, is very bad. But I know that it *can* be good – very good. I am proud to have worked in residential homes, and I know a lot of other people who feel the same. However, the general view – in which there is a dearth of vision – that residential care can never be a positive choice is formed by the bad experience of workers and residents being exploited by people who have neither lived nor worked in residential care.

The politics of residential care

The idea of living a creative and stimulating communal life (or period of life) in anything other than a 'real' family group is rejected as unnatural and inevitably institutionalising. Yet we find that a good proportion of policy makers, especially at central government level, had themselves been sent away to school and persist in doing the same to their children. Presumably, in their view, only some residential institutions are bad for people and it appears that class, culture and wealth denote which are bad and which are good.

Those establishments which house those considered to be the old, the poor, the sick, the needy, the mad and the bad cannot by definition be *chosen* as home because they are defined as places of last resort, dispensing treatment, incarceration or punishment. They inevitably become places for outcasts, places in which people are 'put away'. The possibility that such people may be able to live a creative communal life in the accommodation to which they have been consigned is experienced as a threat. Such success questions received opinion about what constitutes family life and thus challenges the proclaimed values of our society. The majority of households and families are not the neat two parents and child(ren) configuration portrayed in this constricting, conventional and somewhat mythical picture of the family.

Those residential communities which succeed in establishing themselves as strong and self-sufficient are more prone to attack and possible closure than the weak and compliant. And yet it is just such a development – the self-empowerment of users and workers – which I am recommending in this book. Of course, the policy and public intentions of all bodies which own and manage residential services are that they should be empowering places in which to live; at the same time, the effects of organisational domination ensure that they are not.

Strong, vibrant residential communities are perceived to be dangerous because they undermine a society which is based on competition and individual achievement, and on politically propagated 'family values'. Weak residential institutions serve to confirm the worthlessness of a large section of a hierarchical and selfish society, and ensure that those people at the bottom of the heap neither climb it nor demolish it.

Example 9.1   Charity and politics in a children's home

In common with many other residential homes, at Frogmore we used to receive free tickets to charity performances. These were arranged by a well-known show business charity which also specialised in plastering its name on the sides of minibuses. The shows themselves usually appealed to only a small number of the children and young people living at Frogmore. The audiences for these special performances were often people from other homes and welfare organisations. Everyone was given balloons and sweets, and expected to look suitably grateful while they had their photos taken. Most of the residents preferred to keep away from this sort of exploitation and belittlement but we (the staff) never stood in the way of anyone who wanted to go.

I, as head, was phoned one day by the local organiser of this charity, a popular comedy actor. She was concerned that the take-up of free tickets from Frogmore had dwindled so dramatically while other homes in the borough were only too pleased to 'send' their children. I explained the reasons – as acceptably as I could. The organiser exploded with anger and indignation. She inferred from my careful explanation that the children were being gravely misled and felt themselves to be somehow 'above' accepting the charitable gifts and services for which she undoubtedly worked so hard. She went on to accuse me and my colleagues of being 'communists' (as if that was inevitably an insult) and told me she would institute an enquiry into our practice and morals.

I have always thought of this small incident as a nice illustration of the part which receivers of charity and welfare are supposed to play, and of what happens – the deep disturbance caused – when they won't play it. Residents who have a high opinion of themselves, and residential homes which encourage such aspirations, are dangerous misfits in a society constructed on inequality.

Despite their professed ideals, Labour local authorities have not had a noticeably better record of running residential services. There is no instance, to my knowledge, of a Labour council encouraging and supporting the democratic and empowering experience of living and working in residential care. They have suppressed attempts to enable their homes to become places where users and workers take control.

The costs of residential care

The public perception of residential care is cynically manipulated to reject this form of social service on the grounds of cost. Yet it has repeatedly been shown to be cheaper for someone who needs constant care to live in a residential care home than to have the same services brought to their own home (Boyd 1992). Disabled adults have found themselves terribly institutionalised in their own homes, unable to do anything for themselves, immobile and isolated, while a succession of care services are 'delivered' to maintain them 'in the community'.

The cost of public provision has been inflated to bolster the argument for privatising care. Government policies have made local authority residential care very expensive to run – by withholding financial support for residents of council homes while providing extra support to those using private and voluntary homes. The allocation of community care funds will continue this situation by preventing extra financial support of local authority homes while permitting the funding of residents in private and voluntary care homes.

It is clearly cheapest of all – and safer – for the managing authority not to run residential homes and schools at all, but at the same time not to provide an adequate level of support to people in their own homes and ordinary schools. Some local authorities have attempted to get rid of whole sections of residential services. (While Warwickshire closed all their children's homes in the 1980s the county still sent children to residential homes and schools elsewhere; between thirty and forty of them went to Castle Hill in Shropshire where, in 1991, the headteacher was found guilty of raping and abusing children over an eight-year period and sentenced to twelve years in prison.) The government has been willing to pay the private sector to do the work rather than to pay local authorities for the same service.

Government policy has encouraged the huge expansion of private residential care, particularly for older people. Many of those homes which accept residents funded by income support provide minimal care: in spite of the requirements of inspection and registration, homes are often under-staffed by untrained and low-paid workers; too many bedrooms are shared; food and hygiene are often inadequate. Residential care on this basis cannot be a 'positive choice' and remains a last resort in spite of government protestations to the contrary.

This is part of a continuing and sustained attempt to push caring back into the home (which is frequently referred to as the 'community') and re-engage women (mostly) in unpaid and unsupported caring for dependent people. Even if the family cannot cope, it is still low-paid or voluntary workers who are expected to do the caring (again nearly always women). Since in the public and much of the professional view, residential care does not qualify as care in the community, it becomes the shameful last resort – out of the community, 'put away'.

Residential care is part of community care

Residential care is usually the fullest form of provision on a continuum of care which may start with a morning's attendance at a day centre or a once a week visit from a home help. It seems obvious that the day centre and the base for the home help should be in the same place as the flatlet which a person may need in five or ten years time. And these resources must be close by her present home, that is, local, to maximize their usefulness and accessibility. It should be possible for the home help (or community care worker) to be part of the same team which will provide the day or residential care if the person's need for support increases.

Similarly, most children in need of residential care, for whatever reasons, should be able to get that care close to home from people who are working in their own community. These people may work with a child in her own home, with her family and in the residential home.

Moreover, it seems desirable to me that a person's age or particular need or disability, or reason for being to some extent dependent on a social service, should not dictate whether that person goes to an old people's home, or a home for physically disabled people or for people with learning difficulties or even a children's home. Of course, some people may choose to go to a home which specialises in accommodating and caring for people like them, just as some older people choose to live in areas or sheltered housing developments that are exclusively occupied by pensioners. But at the moment there is no choice.

Reflecting the diversity of the community

If residential homes are part of the community they should be for anyone who needs them and chooses them. Their population of residents and outside users and staff should be a true reflection of the community within which they are set and of which they are part.

I think this philosophy particularly applies to local authority establishments. We could leave the specialist homes to the private and voluntary sector so that people have a genuine range of options from which to make a choice. I know some people *would* prefer to be exclusively with their own age group or with others having the same disability. Let those people choose a home where people are segregated like this (there should be no shortage of choice since nearly every place is like that at the moment) and let us start creating houses and larger centres where a whole mixture of people can live together if they choose.

Of course, it is not good to be the first and only person of your age to be living in a place which has traditionally accommodated, say, older people. Nor is it good to be the only Black person in an otherwise all-White resident population. It is important that all users, resident or non-resident, have a sense of belonging and welcome (Chapters 3 and 5) and we should avoid leaving people in a weak, vulnerable and isolated situation, especially when they may be feeling that already. Broadening the range of residents using a home or community care centre must be done with great care so that people are not further marginalised within the establishment.

Spreading ownership and control

The immediate future is likely to bring continued encouragement and pressure to move residential services into more diversified ownership and control. Local authorities are using this as an opportunity to experiment and cooperate with other organisations.

The fact that homes have been owned and run by a local authority has far from ensured their efficacy in policy implementation; indeed, it may sometimes seem to guarantee the opposite. There is nothing essentially good or politically correct (nor bad nor politically incorrect) about public ownership. It is destructive when it imposes the bureaucratic and hierarchical control so inimical to a personal care service. User control, worker democracy and equal opportunities may be much more likely to flourish in more independent and flexible organisations which are neither run for profit nor have the burdens of a large bureaucracy to contend with, but have clear aims to achieve the implementation of publicly declared principles (the primary task).

It is quite possible for local authorities to support the foundation of such independent organisations. It is also feasible that existing homes could be transformed into more independent, helpful and democratic institutions and still remain part of social services departments. It is not important who owns such establishments but only that they provide a high-quality service.

If residential services are to become a positive choice they will take a central role in the provision of a social service. Throughout the history of social services departments, and their forerunners the separate Children's and Welfare Departments, residential care has been the service taking the highest proportion of the budget but at the same time being accorded a low status and a peripheral position in organisational priorities. These were services which departments had to run but took little pride in running. It is rare for any organisation to build up a long and good reputation for running the best residential provision – of any sort. Even when a particular home has stood out for its excellence, it is not usual for the organisation of which it is part to recognise and promote this excellence. Much innovation in residential care is consequently shortlived, depending almost exclusively on the unappreciated and unsupported energy and ideas of insiders – staff and residents.

For this reason, amongst others cited above, it is not surprising that most large organisations, both public and voluntary, have been keen to hive off their residential provision. Residential care homes and centres *are* difficult to run successfully – as this book is at pains to point out. They are risky to run, principally because they accommodate people who for various reasons cannot live in their own homes. They bring apparently intractable problems with them – and the mixture of major personal, social and psychological problems, of severe mental health problems and various disabilities is threatening to any organisation. As seen in Chapter 6, the common organisational responses are defensive: to control, to isolate, to deny, to push away, to render less threatening.

If, however, we could bring residential care, with its more concentrated and dramatic requirements for social work, right into the centre of social service provision; if we could see it as integrated with the rest of the service, and with health and educational services as well; if we could view it as being simply the most concentrated and intensive form of social service – though part and parcel of all the other services – then we would provide residential care most economically, efficiently and effectively.

Example 9.2   Acre Lane Community Care Centre: a vision of the future

Acre Lane Community Care Centre is a large building on a busy road in an inner city area. People come and go all day and well into the evening.

On your first visit to the centre you would be unlikely to know of all the activities and services which it offers. Perhaps you went to a social event held by a club you belong to, or you went for some advice on benefits (a service advertised outside). You wouldn't realise that quite a lot of people live in the building because you didn't see any signs of residential accommodation. In fact, some of the flats are quite separate from the main building and have their own entrances.

If you have lived in the area for some time, you would be much more familiar with the Community Care Centre or, as some people call it, Acre Lane Centre. Others, who have known it for many years, call it 'the home' – a name that signifies one of its main functions and recalls its previous history. It used to be a home for senior citizens, with a day centre and sheltered flats attached. In those days, institutionalised and reeking of urine and disinfectant, it was shunned by local people. The place is now transformed.

Most people in the locality have had or will have something to do with the centre at some time in their lives. Many of the local services are run from there. The council owns the building and funds some of the services. The health authority fund and run other services like chiropody. A number of local voluntary organisations and even a building society and a large supermarket chain are involved. The building society provides a banking service two mornings a week, specially tailored to residents and disabled people in the locality but open to anyone. And the supermarket chain, who have a large store nearby, shares in the running of a nursery at which their own employees can use up to half the places.

People of all ages, female and male, Black and White, of different physical and intellectual abilities – they all use this building. Local councillors give regular surgeries there, as do some doctors, opticians and dentists. There are adult education classes, children's dance classes on a Saturday morning and regular meetings of the local gardening club, whose members look after the garden and help with window boxes and indoor plants throughout the public areas of the building. There is a parents' and toddlers' One O'Clock Club and a weekly Dominoes club run by Caribbean elders. Sometimes, on a Saturday afternoon, a wedding reception is held in the hall and there is a regular programme of plays, music and other entertainment on Thursday evenings. People who go to one event or use one of the services often find themselves returning and getting involved with something else which is going on. Commonly, people receive help and support in one way and give in another.

The building has an average of fifty people living in it. There are two large, three-bedroomed family flats where children, with or without their parents, can be accommodated.

Another part of the building accommodates mostly single people, of all ages from young adults to pensioners. They have their own rooms with a small bathroom en suite, and share a large kitchen, dining and sitting rooms.

On the floor above, another eight very dependent people, who need constant physical assistance with most aspects of daily living, have their own flatlets with bathrooms and toilets (giving easy wheelchair access) and a small food preparation area. They too have a large communal kitchen, dining room and sitting room. Two of these flatlets are for short-term and respite care.

On another floor, where the rooms do not have the advantage of en-suite bathrooms, live people who are usually fairly physically fit but need constant support from staff to maintain the pattern and purpose of their lives.

Daily life and staff help are different in all these separate parts of the building, and change according to the needs of particular residents, but there is no rigid barrier of demarcation according to age or disability which decides which flat or group a person is to live in. Sometimes a person who has Alzheimer's Disease may be happier and thrive better living with other people who are mostly very alert and comprehensible, whereas another person in a similar position may indicate she is happier and more comfortable living with a small group of similarly disabled people.

In addition, there are the separate and self-contained flats which have direct-call systems to staff in the centre so that the tenants can summon help when they require it. All of these tenants need accommodation which is very close to assistance, and they arrange for regular help with any daily living activity which they cannot manage on their own, for instance, getting up and going to bed.

The many uses and complexities of many large buildings are not evident to visitors or even those who live or work in one part of the place. So although the residential part of the Community Care Centre is not immediately apparent to the casual or occasional caller, it would not be long before you met residents or tenants of the Centre, the people who live in the building. If you then got to know them a bit, and they you, you might discover that they lived there. But this discovery would not mark them off from you or anyone else who lived in the same road or round the corner from the Centre. You would not meet them as residents but as fellow users of the Centre, as neighbours, as customers of the building society. It is likely that many other visitors to the Centre would have similar needs or disabilities to those who are resident. Nor will it be obvious who are staff and who are users. People who work at the Centre are likely to be users in some way and most people who use the Centre will make some sort of contribution. (For example, two of the pensioners living in the flats are working with children from a nearby school on a local history project. They've called it Sheep in Acre Lane, because one of the old people remembers sheep being driven to market down Acre Lane.)

There are a minibus and a taxi (an old cab which is adapted for wheelchair transport), for which the community transport committee raised the money and now maintains. The vehicles are in constant use by many different organisations and groups and they are serviced by the local garage in Acre Lane at which one of the residents works. While the community transport is run as a charity for financial reasons, there is nothing charitable about the style of this transport; the residents, staff and local community are clear that it was they who raised the money and who keep this vital service going, and there is great pride in seeing the minibus and taxi out and about.

At the front of the building a large sign names the Centre and a noticeboard advertises all sorts of different events and services going on in the building and in the area around. The mixed sponsorship and funding is made quite clear. The council seem to have no qualms about themselves appearing on the same board as various voluntary and commercial organisations.

There is no longer a separate social services or home care office. The social workers and the people who used to be home helps, even the meals-on-wheels service, are all run from the Acre Lane Centre. The staff are part of the Community Care team and so are the staff of the residential units. So are the child protection workers and the foster care support workers. The building and the manner in which it is run and the message it conveys all demonstrate that this is a community resource open to everyone who needs it and who wishes to participate in or make a contribution to its activities.

A Community Care service

There are, of course, some things which the Centre does not and cannot do. It is different from all the other community care centres in the borough. The Acre Lane Centre is one of the largest buildings of its type, with the most diverse services and activities. Some of the smaller homes have also been gradually converted into multipurpose centres but do not accommodate so many people. Some cannot yet take children and families, and others are not suitable for older people who are physically disabled (there is no room to provide en-suite bathrooms).

The local authority still needs to make provision for some specially needy, ill or disabled people, for instance, some very emotionally disturbed children, or some people with such a profound mental disability that they have not attained any apparent communication with others: people who have a right to very specialised care, education and training. Sometimes the other larger community care centres may be able to provide for one or two such people, but the borough has also taken care to develop smaller community care centres which specialise in care for people with particular needs. Instead of sending people away from their area they stay in the borough and these small centres are also well connected in their local community. The same principles of community involvement and responsibility apply to the smaller special centres as to the larger ones.

Some of the centres are leased from the council by housing associations, or voluntary care organisations who are then paid by the council to provide services. A couple of centres are owned by voluntary organisations. Several operate from a number of buildings in a small area but are seen and used as a coordinated and comprehensive local service. But every centre has to demonstrate that it is managed by and for its users and the local community. Each centre has its own way of working which has grown up as the centre has developed. What is needed and works in one locality is not necessarily suitable in another. The choices about what to fund and what services to provide are made by local people, users, staff, carers and volunteers.

The centres are complex organisations but self-governing and self-managing. There is a centre manager whose job is less to direct than to coordinate. She is an expert in managing cooperation and collaboration. There are many different teams of workers in the place but all of them have a minimum of hierarchy – just a team leader with all other team members capable of taking their turns at managing the team. There is not a large gap in pay between the care workers (who are comparatively well paid), managers and team leaders. They all bear in mind that their team provides a service which is part of and linked with all the other services. They have to work cooperatively and flexibly for the community care centre to succeed. A lot of the staff live locally and use the centre themselves. Being a user of community care is not a demeaning or passive experience. Being a community care worker is a job with public respect but also immediate and close public scrutiny.

Catering, domestic and maintenance staff, whose main responsibilities are to provide good food and to keep the centre's fabric and equipment clean and fit for its purpose, are also very prominent and valued members of their teams. They are expected to take part in the full activities of the centre, providing social and emotional support for users at the same time as doing ordinary and important practical jobs. Everyone (users and workers of all grades), is expected to participate in the domestic tasks of the place. If something needs cleaning up urgently, or a lavatory is dirty, you are just as likely to see the centre coordinator with a mop in her hand as you are to see a member of one of the care teams.

The administrative staff are of vital importance in the place. The finances are complicated and ever changing. But there is a commitment to open and non-bureaucratic administration. The accounts are published (and audited of course) and cost effectiveness is always an issue. However, since people are privy to all the financial information, and can be involved with making difficult financial decisions, some of the more expensive care is not

> begrudged but is a matter of pride and achievement, and will in any case attract special extra local and central government and charitable funds.
>
> The local authority continues to run centrally controlled services alongside the community care centres but has reduced or converted them as the centres begin to take their place for statutory services. The conversion will take some years. The authority still maintains some central support services but even these are modelled on a mixture of user, worker, and elected democratic management.

These community care centres may sound a nightmare of chaotic complexity, especially to people in large organisations where everything has been administered and controlled from the centre. However, if we consider the present arrangements for social services and residential care it is clear that the large bureaucratic departments fail to provide responsive and effective services. Where those services do exist in a suitable form, it is in spite of rather than because of the control and administrative complexity imposed by the central organisation.

EXPLOITING THE BANDWAGON OF SUPERFICIAL CHANGE

One of the lessons of trades union and local politics since 1979 is that pitched battles do not win wars for the weaker side. When residential workers took widespread industrial action in 1984, demanding better pay and conditions, they separated themselves from residents – users – and their families. They lost their most potent allies. Local authorities took the opportunity to close residential establishments, the pace of privatisation was hastened and residential workers gained very little of what they were seeking. In spite of regular scandals and enquiries, in spite of reports, policy and legislation there has been little overall improvement in residential services.

Amongst the mass of much trumpeted but largely superficial changes are many openings for deeper changes and improvements. A new philosophy of business and government – to reduce the burden of the centre and to give more responsibility and scope to local services – often appears to be contradicted by their actions, yet it is a philosophy which suits attempts to build more democratic and autonomous services. There are many elements of recent legislation and policy which can be used to encourage a more flexible and independent approach to social service provision. The idea of cost centres, where the budget is devolved and localised, was not primarily intended to increase local democratic control of services but simply to encourage more financial stringency and individual responsibility. However, used imaginatively and creatively, devolving the budget is an essential part of giving users control over their own lives in residence. Similarly, the concept of 'community care' has in it the seeds of community development and the integration of all social services, including residential care. (The current trend is the segregation of services. Policy makers have scapegoated 'genericism' as the great mistake of the past twenty years rather than detecting a more fundamental flaw in the organisation and politics of social service.)

For the sort of developments of local community care centres that I sketch above to become a reality there has to be a major change in policy and practice from the centre (local and national). But the opportunities for change are already open. There has been much talk about 'resource centres' multipurpose residential and day care establishments. There has even been some action. Sheffield set up what it called EPSUs – Elderly Persons' Service Units – in the early 1980s. Kent, a local authority often in the forefront of new developments, have been establishing their Linked Service Centres, intended to provide a comprehensive service to pensioners. Resource centres have been operating all over the country for some years. Some, despite their new name, did not change their operation in any significant way, but others have become much more connected to their local communities and have opened themselves up.

The resource centre idea has really worked where local authorities have been willing and able to relinquish their control. The residents, staff and other users of a local centre will agitate for self-management and self-determination, and the central managers and elected members who see this as an exciting and productive development will be those who are able to let go. However, those who simply see a threat (which it is) to their highly paid and powerful positions will fight tooth and nail to prevent this concept of community care, while at the same time braying the rhetoric of user empowerment.

A major barrier to these exciting changes is the incorporation of large cohorts of managers and administrators into centralist organisations. Thousands of people are in the way: people who spend their time being important, speaking in acronyms and jargon, writing reports and making bids; people who are mesmerised by the new managerial and financial language of social care, which really does not have anything to do with the wellbeing of users or staff, and is all about petty ambition, power and money.

The radical change needed to liberate residential centres will be a slow process, taking many years. It will require directors of social service organisations, both public and voluntary, who are prepared to change the nature of their jobs and hand back power to users, to the workforce and to local people. Similarly, councils and management committees must relinquish their authoritarian role. True community care in this sense is not an administrative and managerial convenience: it is a social revolution. However, just as the people at the top have never been able to make deep changes in society without the initiative and revolutionary energy of the people, nor will even the most wellmeaning of them achieve a genuine transfer of power in social services unless there are people willing and able to take power for themselves. At all levels we share responsibility for achieving changes. At the top, politicians and senior managers must let go and encourage every initiative from the users and workforce, who for their part must take the initiative and create their own popular institutions.

It is not expected that social services organisations of any sort, whether in the public, private or voluntary sectors, will make these changes without a struggle. We are faced with organisations which have a record of changing only when forced to do so. The fundamental changes I envisage will be led by the determination of users and workers to break out of the straightjackets imposed on them by all forms of government and organisation, whether it be under the guise of 'value for money', or 'quality'. or 'customer care', or even 'community care', all of which boil down to an imposition of new systems and procedures designed to make organisations look good rather than give a good service. However, we can use these empty policy proclamations in conjunction with the reports on which they are based to initiate the radical changes which we know are needed at the level of where the service is used and given. Every government report, enquiry and White Paper, every pronouncement from the great and the good has something of value in it to be used as a channel for change. (Of course, some such publications *are* intended to directly influence government legislation and to fuel the fundamental changes which we want – for example, the 1988 *Wagner Report*).

Example 9.3 Taking the initiative and making practical changes

At Inglewood in the early 1980s we were faced with a building containing eight four-bedded rooms, sixteen double and fifty-six single bedrooms, designed to accommodate 120 people. We were determined to get rid of the four-bedded rooms. Sharing with one other person, unless by choice, was bad enough; being forced to share with three was disgraceful. No-one could defend this state of affairs as good practice and it had to be changed.

We were all (residents and staff) involved in making plans for the conversion of the home to smaller units – to group living. Opinions were widely canvassed and there was an officially constituted planning group which included residents, staff and outsiders. The converted accommodation would reduce the overall maximum resident population to eighty-seven.

All the four-bedded rooms would be converted to doubles or to communal rooms like dining rooms, and the original double-bedded rooms would remain as they were. But these plans which we were making would not be implemented for at least two years and meanwhile residents were forced to share.

Our immediate objective was to get rid of the four-bedded rooms and reduce the overall numbers in the building. Obviously, one way we did this was by offering people who slept in four-bedded rooms the option of other rooms as soon as they became vacant. We then removed the beds from the multi-occupied rooms until they became double rooms.

Because a reduction in numbers had not yet been agreed by the council, we were not 'allowed' to do this. So I took the first opportunity to implicate the new vice-chair of the social services committee by inviting him to Inglewood and showing him what we were doing. In spite of the objections and warnings of the assistant director of social services who accompanied him, he could do little but agree with our actions. To some extent he was tricked into compliance but since I had heard him state very clearly that 'This council will not condone older people being forced to share rooms', that was enough for me.

Neither he nor the assistant director could very well ask to have the beds replaced since they knew that I would remind them of the occasion when the committee vice-chair had agreed with what we had done. If necessary, I would simply have refused to comply with such a request on the grounds that it was bad practice with which I could not collude. It would have been foolish to attempt to discipline me over such a matter.

That was our first move in taking the responsibility and initiative to reduce numbers and rid the place of multi-occupied rooms. Our next step was to draw up the plans for the new units. I knew that the four-bedded rooms could not be converted into two viable double-bedded rooms, but they appeared as such on the plans. I let that go because I knew that when the conversion had been done we would use the rooms as two, better-sized singles with space for someone to manoeuvre a wheelchair and have an armchair in the room. That is what subsequently happened. I recently spent some time with one of the people who has been living in one of these converted rooms (a contributor to Chapter 8). She is a wheelchair user in her nineties who has arranged the room as she wants it but, even so, there is barely space for all her requirements. Looking back, it seems preposterous that this room was planned to accommodate two people.

We continued to resist the compulsory sharing of rooms, and in 1984 (two years after we had initiated our reforms at Inglewood) we received the official backing we required. In that year, the standards by which private and voluntary residential care homes should be run were set out in *Home Life* (Centre for Policy on Ageing 1984). Our council was responsible for enforcing these standards, included in which was the firm statement (on page 64): 'It is recommended that residents in long-term care should have their own rooms, unless they prefer otherwise.'

This on-the-ground implementation of good practice was fought, resisted, undermined, ignored and sabotaged by senior managers and councillors for several more years, in spite of their continued empty proclamations about residents' rights and improving practice, and the clear recommendations set out in *Home Life*. I understand that this local authority has now, at last, accepted the principle in practice, and no-one is compelled to share a room in any of the homes it runs. Many other managing organisations continue to ignore the principle and condone the bad practice.

That is just one example of how changes can be led and sustained by the actions of workers and users, and of how our local initiatives do make a contribution to wider progressive practice. It is essential to enlist every available source of help. Amongst the resistant and oppressive array of managers and committee members there will be some people who *are* committed to good practice and who are willing to fight with you if you lead the way. Occasionally, you will find allies at the very top of organisations who will take considerable risks in supporting user and worker initiatives.

It is noticeable that the less power an individual or a group proposing change has, the more radical the proposals can be. The nearer the proposals come to legislation or publicly declared policy the more watered-down, discretionary and woolly become the proposals. In the process of policy formulation, all the power holders have their say, and since there are no radical changes which do not involve a shift in power, policy usually emerges in a form which maintains the original power relationships.

Our job in residential work is to shift power relationships – starting with our own – towards user power. In doing so we will ally ourselves directly and unequivocally with users and will always be unpopular with the 'powers that be'. 'Liberating institutions' is a deliberately ambiguous phrase. I believe that existing institutions require collective vision and commitment, creativity and cunning, militancy and energy (some of the qualities we bring to direct work with people) to transform them from centres of oppression into places of liberation and life. It can be done.

Appendix 1

The learning basket

The Learning Basket is a metaphor for learning together. I use this at the beginning of most training and development work.

When I join a group of people to learn or to participate in some change, I bring with me my experience, knowledge, ideas, feelings, principles, my stories, words and pictures. I usually bring some sort of bag or case which contains books and papers, Blu-tack, markers and other bits and pieces to use in the work. But this bag cannot contain all my knowledge and experience and all the other things I listed. When I come to meet with the group it is as if I also bring a learning basket which contains all these other intangible goods. I draw a basket:

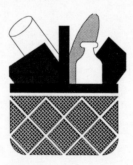

Figure A1   The learning basket

Everyone brings a learning basket. Our baskets contain different things and different combinations of things. Some people will have more experience of the work than others; some more formal education or training; everyone will have a way of thinking or a belief or an idea which no-one else has.

If I give you something from my basket – if I tell you one of my ideas – I still have it after I have given it away. In fact, it may well be better, more developed, more alive because in the process of giving it to you, we discussed it; I had another look at it; I re-evaluated it; I heard what you had to say about it; I added one of your ideas to it.

Sometimes I look in my basket and produce something which I have been carrying around for a long time, and only when I bring it out into the light of day do I realise it has been a burden and a nuisance to me. Other people help me to look at this and I decide to leave it behind. I don't have to carry it around any more.

I will also come with space in my basket – my ignorance of some topics, my lack of experience in some areas, my dearth of ideas in others – but my space is someone else's opportunity. My ignorance is an opening for someone with knowledge. She can produce her knowledge; in accepting it from her I can help to refine it, to make it understandable; I can apply it to my own experience and it becomes my knowledge.

At the bottom of my basket I have packages which have been there for years, tightly tied up. I know they are there and yet I forget them. I know they affect me, yet I leave them alone. Something may happen for me in this group, on this course, which may encourage me to take the chance and have a look inside. I will discover things which are both difficult and liberating. I choose which packages to open and which to leave wrapped up, or whether I open any at all.

The process of learning together is a process of mutual discovery, free exchange and gaining something new.

Appendix 2

Change

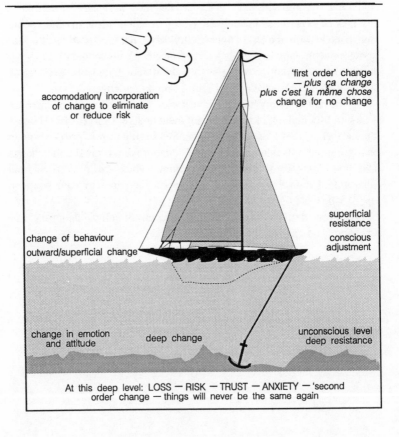

Figure A2   An image and some ideas about different levels of change
and resistance to change

Risk and trust – a leader in change must experience and demonstrate her or his own deep involvement, willingness to take risks and the capacity to trust. Don't simply ask others to work at this level – they won't if you don't.

UNDERSTANDING LOSS AND CHANGE: LOSS IS CHANGE/CHANGE IS LOSS

Superficial changes need to be strategically and conceptually connected with deep, long term changes. Your vision of change must be FULLY SHARED.

Superficial resistance can sometimes provide a cover and a means for deep change – don't assume that it is deep resistance. Be careful not to attack superficial resistance; give people time, room and support in their process of change.

You can't make people change but you can make them appear to change. Be wary of superficial, quick change – it is likely to cover deep resistance. Try to work at both levels at the same time – on the surface and with the emotional anchors.

Apply the same analysis to yourself as you do to others. Respect your loss of old ways, your resistance to new ones – that respect will enable you to change.

Models, images and cultures of organisations, establishments, units, homes and teams

Remember that even in just a short visit to an establishment you are picking up masses of information. Be alive to all the evidence around you, through eyes, nose, ears, touch, feel, heart, brain and soul, with your antennae vibrating! In nearly every place there are *good* and *bad* things – don't miss the bad, and don't be blinded by the good or by the 'presentation' so that you miss what is really going on under the surface. Always imagine what it would be like to be one of the users of this service.

SOME OF THE QUESTIONS YOU MIGHT ASK YOURSELF

A   *What physical impression does this organisation create?*

1   What immediate impression do you have on approaching, gaining admission, and within five minutes of entering?
2   What can you gather from other simple physical signs – keys, toilets, locked doors, notices, decoration, furniture, food, the clothes people wear, the smell, who goes into which rooms?
3   If this organisation was an animal (tree, machine, piece of furniture, feature of the landscape or weather, etc) what sort would it be?
4   What are the images and metaphors which come to your mind? And which have you heard people in the place using – a bog, a maze, a giant machine, a shit-heap, a feather bed, a factory farm, a warehouse, a greenhouse, a comfy armchair, a family, a holiday camp? And what do they *mean*?
5   How/what does this place make you *feel*?

B   *What is the place here for? What is its primary task?*

1   Is that simply stated for all to see? How else is it expressed?

2 Is there a 'What ought to happen' and a 'What does happen'? Are they connected or is the gap too great?
3 What beliefs and values are evident – on the surface? Beneath the surface?
4 What are the dos and don'ts?

C   What does the language tell you – the everyday talk – the common words and phrases?

1 What do people call each other?
2 What titles are used?
3 What is the history? What are the stories, myths and legends? Are there ghosts? What messages do the stories convey?
4 Do people say 'We, our, us' or do they say '*my* staff', '*my* residents', '*my* home'?

D   How do people get together and talk?

1 How else do they communicate?
2 What issues predominate?
3 How 'open' is communication?
4 What are the topics of informal communication?
5 What are the jokes and gossip?
6 How are visitors introduced, and who to?

E   What is the structure/hierarchy?

1 Who is where in it? Where are the users?
2 Is there any evidence of Equality of Opportunity – the policy? the practice?
3 Think about this for Race, Gender, Age, Disability, Sexuality and other areas of discrimination. For instance, can you see what you would genuinely call anti-racist practice in any area of the organisation's functioning?

F   Who do you think are the three most influential people?

How do they express the essential character of the organisation?

G   What are the subcultures?

1   Are they in harmony or conflict?
2   What purpose do they serve for their members/for the organisation?

(This list of questions has been built up and adapted from 'Understanding the Culture of Your Organisation', an exercise in *Creative Organisation Theory*, Morgan 1989.)

Bibliography

This bibliography contains all those books and articles referred to in the text. In addition I have included a wide range of books which have influenced my thinking and writing. It is not intended to be a comprehensive bibliography of residential care.

Ahmed, B. (1990) *Black Perspective in Social Work*, Birmingham: Venture Press.
Atherton, J. (1986) *Professional Supervision in Group Care*, London: Tavistock.
Atherton, J. (1989) *Interpreting Residential Life*, London: Tavistock/Routledge.
Axline, V. (1972) *Dibs; In Search of Self*, Harmondsworth: Penguin.
Beedell, C. (1970) *Residential Life with Children*, London: Routledge and Kegan Paul.
Benson, J. (1987) *Working More Creatively with Groups*, London: Tavistock.
Bion, W. (1968, 1980) *Experiences in Groups*, London: Tavistock.
Bowlby, J. (1991) *The Making and Breaking of Affectional Bonds*, London: Tavistock/Routledge.
Boyd, P. (1992) 'What price care in the community', *Care Weekly*, July 16.
Brearley, C. (1990) *Working in Residential Homes for Elderly People*, London: Tavistock/Routledge.
Brook, E. and Davis, A. (eds) (1985) *Women, the Family and Social Work*, London: Tavistock.
Brown, A. and Clough, R. (eds) (1989) *Groups and Groupings*, London: Tavistock/Routledge.
Brown, D. and Peddar, J. (1979) *Introduction to Psychotherapy*, London: Tavistock.
Burn, M. (1956) *Mr Lyward's Answer*, London: Hamish Hamilton.
Burton, J. (1988) 'Residential care: change from the inside' (A series of five articles), *Social Work Today*, January 28 – March 10.
Burton, J. (1989a) 'Making it work: group living in residential care', 'Can feelings be part of the job?' 'Keeping faith in desperate times', 'Value of vision: making it work' (A series of four articles), *Social Work Today*, April 6 – May 18.
Burton, J. (1989b) 'Institutional change and group action: the significance and influence of groups in developing new residential services for older people', in Brown, A. and Clough, R. (eds) *Groups and Groupings*, London: Tavistock/Routledge.

Burton, J. (1989c) 'Quite right, Mrs Smith, you're not a cupboard', *Care Weekly*, June 30.

Burton, J. (1990a) 'When pilfering the sardines is a red herring', *Care Weekly*, May 25.

Burton, J. (1990b) 'Speaking for ourselves', 'Rule from the inside out', 'Plugging into user power' (A series of three articles), *Care Weekly*, July 13 – 27.

Burton, J. (1991a) 'Drawing chalk circles', *Community Care*, July 6.

Burton, J. (1991b) 'Doing it by the book', *Social Work Today*, July 25.

Centre for Policy on Ageing (1984) *Home Life: a Code of Practice for Residential Care* London.

Clark, N. (1991) *Managing Personal Learning and Change*, London: McGraw-Hill.

Clough, R. (1981) *Old Age Homes*, London: George Allen and Unwin.

Cockburn, C. (1977) *The Local State*, London: Pluto.

Cohen, S. (1985) *Visions of Social Control*, Cambridge: Polity.

Comfort, A. (1977) *A Good Age*, London: Mitchell Beazley.

Coulshed, V. (1990) *Management in Social Work*, London: Macmillan.

Dainow, S. and Bailey, C. (1990) *Developing Skills with People*, Chichester: Wiley.

Davis, L. (1982) *Residential Care: a Community Resource*, London: Heinemann.

Dearling, A. (1991) *Effective Use of Teambuilding*, Harlow: Longman.

De Board, R. (1978) *The Psychoanalysis of Organisations*, London: Tavistock.

Dennis, F. (1988) *Behind the Frontlines*, London: Gollancz.

Department of Health (1989a) *Caring for People: Community Care in the Next Decade and Beyond*, London: HMSO.

Department of Health (1989b) *Homes Are for Living In*, London: HMSO.

Department of Health (1991) *Children in the Public Care (The Utting Report)*, London: HMSO.

Dharamsi, F., Edmonds, G., Filkin, E., Headley, C., Jones, P., Naish, M., Scott, J., Smith, E., Smith, H. and Williams, J. (1979) *Community Work and Caring for Children*, Ilkley: Owen Wells.

Dockar-Drysdale, B. (1968) *Therapy in Child Care*, London: Longman.

Dockar-Drysdale, B. (1973) *Consultation in Child Care*, London: Longman.

Dominelli, L. (1988) *Anti-racist Social Work*, London: Macmillan.

Douglas, R. and Payne, C. (1987) *Learning About Caring* (Four sections), London: National Institute for Social Work.

Douglas, R. and Payne, C. (1988) *Organising for Learning*, London: National Institute for Social Work.

Douglas, R. Ettridge, D., Fearnhead, D., Payne, C., Pugh, D. and Sowter, D. (1988) *Helping People Work Together*, London: National Institute for Social Work.

Douglas, T. (1986) *Group Living*, London: Tavistock.

Douglas, T. (1991) *A Handbook of Common Groupwork Problems*, London: Tavistock/Routledge.

Ford, K. and Hargreaves, S. (1991) *First-line Management: Staff*, Harlow, Longman.

Fryer, P. (1984) *Staying Power: the History of Black People in Britain*, London, Pluto.

Gilroy, P. (1987) *There Ain't No Black in the Union Jack*, London: Hutchinson.

Goffman, E. (1961) *Asylums: Essays on the Social Situation of Mental Patients and Other Inmates*, New York: Doubleday.

Harris, J. and Kelly D. (1991) *Management Skills in Social Care*, Aldershot: Gower.

Hawkins, P. and Shohet, R. (1989) *Supervision in the Helping Professions*, Buckingham: Open University Press.

Hill, S. (1990) *More Than Rice and Peas*, London: The Food Commission.

HMSO (1989) *The Children Act*, London: HMSO.

Houston, G. (1990) *Supervision and Counselling*, London: Gaie Houston.

Illich, I. (1973) *Celebration of Awareness*, Harmondsworth: Penguin.

Jaques, E. (1955) 'Social systems as a defence against persecutory and depressive anxiety', in Klein, M., Heimann, P. and Money-Kyrle, R. (eds) *New Directions in Psychoanalysis*, London: Tavistock.

Jones, H. (1978) *The Residential Community: a Setting for Social Work*, London: Routledge and Kegan Paul.

Jordan, J. (1987) 'Other kinds of dreams'; an interview with June Jordan', *Spare Rib*, November.

Jordan, J. (1989) *Moving towards Home: Political Essays*, London: Virago.

Kent County Council Social Services (1991) *A Guide to the Good Care of Elderly People with Mental Health Difficulties*.

Klein, M. (1959) 'Our adult world and its roots in infancy', *Human Relations* 12: 291–303.

Knapp, M. (1984) *The Economics of Social Care*, London: Macmillan.

Landau, M. and Stout, R. (1979) 'To manage is not to control: or the folly of type II errors', *Public Administration Review*, March/April.

Landry, C., Morley, D., Southwood, R. and Wright, P. (1985) *What a Way to Run a Railroad*, London: Comedia.

Lane, D. (1980) *Staffing Ratios in Residential Establishments*, London: Residential Care Association.

Levi, P. (1987) *Moments of Reprieve*, London: Sphere Books.

Marris, P. (1986) *Loss and Change*, London: Routledge and Kegan Paul.

Martin, S. (1983) *Managing without Managers*, London: Sage.

Menzies, I. (1970) *The Functioning of Social Systems as a Defence against Anxiety*, Tavistock Pamphlet No. 3, London: Tavistock.

Menzies Lyth, I. (1988) *Containing Anxiety in Institutions*, London: Free Association Books.

Menzies Lyth, I. (1989) *The Dynamics of the Social*, London: Free Association Books.

Morgan, G. (1986) *Images of Organization*, London: Sage.

Morgan, G. (1989) *Creative Organisation Theory*, London: Sage.

Moss, M. (1991) 'Making ideal homes', *Community Care*, August 1.

Mulgen, G. (1988) 'The power of the weak', *Marxism Today*, December.

Murphy, E. (1991) *After the Asylums; Community Care for People with a Mental Illness*, London: Faber and Faber.

NISW/HMSO (1988) *A Positive Choice (The Wagner Report)*, London: National Institute for Social Work/HMSO.

Parkes, C. (1971) 'Psycho-social transitions: a field for study', *Social Science and Medicine* Vol. 5, 101–15.

Payne, C. (1989) *Better Services for Older People*, London: National Institute for Social Work.

Pedlar, M. and Boydell, T. (1985) *Managing Yourself*, London: Fontana.

Pedlar, M., Burgoyne, J. and Boydell, T. (1986) *A Manager's Guide to Self-development*, London: McGraw-Hill.

Peters, T. (1989) *Thriving on Chaos*, London: Pan.

Phillipson, C. and Walker, A. (eds) (1986) *Ageing and Social Policy*, Aldershot: Gower.

Pick, P. (1981) *Children at Tree Tops: an Example of Creative Residential Care*, London: Residential Care Association.

Reason, P. (1984) 'Is organisation development possible in power cultures?' in Kakabadse, A. and Parker, C. (eds) *Power, Politics, and Organizations: a Behaviour Science View*, Chichester: Wiley.

Redl, F. (1966) *When we deal with Children*, New York: The Free Press.

Redl, F. and Wineman, D. (1965) *Controls from Within*, New York: The Free Press.

Rice, A. (1958) *Productivity and Social Organisations: the Ahmedabad Experiment*, London: Tavistock.

Rose, M. (1990) *Healing Hurt Minds*, London: Routledge.

Salzberger-Wittenberg, I. (1970) *Psycho-analytic Insight and Relationships: a Kleinian Approach*, London: Routledge and Kegan Paul.

Schein, E. (1988) *Process Consultation*, Wokingham: Addison Wesley.

Segal, J. (1985) *Phantasy in Everyday Life*, Harmondsworth: Penguin.

Senior, B. (1989) 'Residential care: what hope for the future?' in Langan, M. and Lee, P. (eds) *Radical Social Work Today*, London: Unwin.

Social Care Association (1980) *Staffing in Residential Homes*, London: Social Care Association.

Staffordshire County Council (1991) *The Pindown Experience and the Protection of Children: the Report of the Staffordshire Childcare Inquiry, 1990*, Stafford: Staffordshire County Council.

Stanton, A. (1989) *Invitation to Self Management*, Ruislip: Dab Hand Press.

Trist, E. and Bamforth, K. (1951) 'Some social and psychological consequences of the longwall method of coal-cutting', *Human Relations* 4 (1): 3 – 38.

Ward, C. (1982) *Anarchy in Action*, London: Freedom Press.

Watt, S. (1992) 'Minimum age call for carers', *Care Weekly*, 20 March, 3.

Williams, A. (1991) *Forbidden Agendas: Strategic Action in Groups*, London: Routledge.

Wills, D. (1971) *Spare the Child*, Harmondsworth: Penguin.

Winnicott, D. W. (1964) *The Child, the Family and the Outside World*, Harmondsworth: Penguin.

Winnicott, D. (1978) *The Family and Individual Development*, London: Tavistock.

Worsley, J. (1989) *Taking Good Care*, Mitcham: Age Concern England.

Worsley, J. (1992) *Good Care Management*, London: Age Concern England.

Index

acceptance 51, 69, 97–8
abuse 56 (*see also* sexual, sexist and racist abuse)
administrative staff 179
admission(s) xiii, 17–19, 34, 42–6, 129, 133, 152, 158, 165, 167
adolescents 62–4, 68
adolescent unit 162–3
African 8
age 191
agenda 104
agreements 116
allegations 60, 63
Alzheimer's disease 116, 177
anger 14, 54, 83, 100, 148
anxiety: defence(s) against 129–43
appointments 37, 84, 149
assessment 43, 49, 130, 136
assistant director 17–18, 183
Atherton, J. 105
attention seeking 29, 165
authority 65, 67–9

baby, babies 10, 47–9, 65, 88, 100
basic care 49, 56
BASW (British Association of Social Workers) 87
bath book 141
bathing 56–8, 138–41
bathroom(s) 99
Beck, Frank 75
bed sores 4–6
bedtime 11, 49, 52–6
Beedell, C. xv, 97
Bion, W. 125

birthdays 122
bisexual 59
Bishop of Southwark 91
Black: children 8, 47; residents 109, 165; staff 33
Bottomley, Virginia 87
Boyd, P 172
boundaries 41, 61, 62, 98, 102, 126, 137, 142, 146–8, 151–2, 158
Brent xiv
Bristol Royal Infirmary xv
Bristol University (and School for Advanced Urban Studies) xv
Brixton xiv
budget 94
buildings 90–1
bureaucracy 35, 78, 133, 136, 143, 151, 174, 180

care assistant(s) 60, 74, 138, 153
care management 141
Castle Hill 172
chairs 92–3
change 15, 24, 34, 75–6, 85–7, 91–2, 118–21, 180–5, 188–9
charity 171
childhood, regression 10
Children Act 134
choice 58, 72, 75, 93–4, 98, 101, 174
Clark, N. 80
clothes 45, 53, 55, 165
Clough, R. xv
Comfort, A. 97
communal life 41, 170
communists 171

community care 172, 173, 178, 181
community care centre 175–80
complaint(s) 139
computer 113
consultant(s) 83, 108, 145, 152–6
contraception 59
control 12, 54, 64–9, 75, 163, 171
cook(s) 101, 109
cooking 16, 100–2, 165
coroner 139
cost(s): of furniture 94; of residential
    care 172–3
cost centres 181
Cotswold Community xv
cricket 9
crisis 36, 39
CSV (Community Service
    Volunteers) xii
culture(s) 34, 93, 95–8, 101–2, 104,
    111, 115, 120
cycling 39

damage 93
death 5, 50, 122, 129
decisions 32, 78–9, 93–4, 102–5,
    121, 133, 152, 158
decoration 93
democracy 21, 104, 174, 180
dependency 88, 168
deputy 85
diary 9, 29, 31, 37–8, 54, 106
Dickson, Alec xii
difficult behaviour 49
director 74
disabled people 24, 70, 96, 164, 167,
    172, 177, 191
disciplinary 137, 140
discrimination 191
Dockar-Drysdale, B. 93
domestic worker(s) 5, 74, 95, 104,
    109, 167, 179
dominoes 176
drugs 54, 158–60, 163
durability 95
duty person 16, 43
dying 4–6

enquiry 140, 180
environment 126

equality 59, 60, 102, 191

family 170; dynamics 89
fantasy 41–2, 46, 50, 80, 83
father 46–8
feedback 126
file(s) 50, 166
fire risks 13–14
flatlets 177
food 44, 49, 78–9, 92, 100–2,
    109–11, 164
football 161
forms 36, 40
Frogmore xiv, 7–13, 90, 92, 131,
    147, 171
furniture 91–5

game(s) 7
garden 16, 176
gender 12, 13, 67, 191
genericism 181
Goffman, E. 129, 132
good experience 47
graffiti 129
grandparent(s) 59, 88; 'streetwise
    grannies' 87
group living 91–2, 99, 183

Hammersmith xiv
Hawkins, P. and Shohet, R. 105
hierarchy 26, 96, 102, 130, 142, 170,
    174, 179, 191
Hill, S. 102
Hindu 122
history 50, 51
HIV 59
hoist(s) 57, 99, 167
holding 12, 66–7
Home Life 184
Homes Are For Living In 90
homosexual 59, 62
hot-water bottle 53
Houston, G. 105–6, 152

incontinence 4–6, 138–9
inequality 96, 171
Inglewood xv, 4, 13–15, 19–21,
    42–6, 90, 103, 132, 182–4
innovation 175

inspection 90, 103, 139–40, 146, 148–50, 172
institutional defences 62, 84, 126–43, 175
institutionalisation 44, 66, 92, 114, 129, 132, 133, 170, 172, 176
Ireland 160

Jaques, E. 125, 129
Jewish 122
job description 28, 80

Kent 181
kitchen(s) 16, 99

LCC 90
Labour 20, 171
Lambeth xv, 4, 20
laundry 131
lavatories 91, 99, 102, 168, 179
law 116, 118
leadership 36, 73–7, 85; roles 77
learning disabilities 19–20, 70, 116, 178
leaving 122
legislation 134
lifting 6, 57
Liverpool 20
lock(s) 99, 130
loss 8, 50

management: democratic 75–7; everyday 24–6; and gender 25–6; parasitic management 37; paternal management 77; reassessment of 73–7
management group 35–7
manager(s) 19, 73, 88–9, 102, 105, 108, 111, 113, 136–8, 145, 150–2, 179, 181, 184; see also Supermanager
managing 15, 124; your own work 39–40
managing time 38–40
meetings: children's 10; community xv, 79, 121, 166; staff 9, 36, 102–5, 118–20, 131; residents' 120–1, 159, 162, 167
menu(s) 110

Menzies, I. 125, 129, 132
Millard, P. 97
mission statement 131
mistakes 8–9, 12, 15, 154
Morgan, G. 192
mothering 48, 165
music 53
Muslim 122–3

natural materials 92
night staff 6, 13, 168
nightmares 52
'No' 84, 86, 143
North Paddington Upper School xii
not giving up 67
notices 116–17
nursery 164

observing children 49
office 17, 36
office hours 137
old people 51, 72
outsider(s) 145–56
'over-involvement' 60

paperwork 136
parenting, and management 85, 87–9
Paris 164
Part III (National Assistance Act) 43
pension book 14
personal care 4–6, 51, 56–8
phantasy 41–2
photographs 95–6
physical diabilities 60
pictures 95–7
'pin-down' 75, 123
planning 20, 34, 57, 104, 110, 123, 134; a shift 16, 55; your own work 38–40, 83, 86
pocket money 162, 163, 165
police 11
policy 134, 138–42
politics 19–21, 170–1
pottery 30
power 25, 33, 75, 80, 143, 184; abuse of 59; letting go of 21–2, 182; personal 25–6
pride 100
principle 32–5

prison xiii, 126, 158
privacy 99
privatising 172
probation hostel xii
procedure(s) 137, 141; manual 140
process 126, 130
promotion 85–6
public and private 98–9
public ownership 174
punishment(s) 52, 64, 68, 116–17
purchasers and providers 134

race 12, 191
racism 47, 96, 102
racist abuse 33
rate capping 20
reception area 98
referral(s) 44, 155
regression 10, 49
relationships 46–52
relatives 92, 94
reliability 28–32
religion 115, 122–3
resentment (of residential workers) 15
residents' power 21
resource centres 181
respite care 94, 177
responsibility 75, 151
restraint 64
review 83, 108–10
rewards, of the job 69–71
Rice, A. 124
risk(s) 44, 58, 64, 66, 88, 131,
    139–42, 153, 169
ritual(s) 55, 114, 121–2
role(s) 45, 48, 79, 85–6, 103, 142
room(s) 6, 73, 91, 93–4, 162
Rose, M. 78
rota(s) 111–14
routines 55, 114–21
rules 114–21, 143, 160

sabotage 73, 113
sanctions 64, 69
scandal(s) 125, 138–41, 144, 180
school xiii, 17, 50, 161–2
security 13, 99, 166
self, managing yourself 24,
    responsibility for 25, use of 66

self-analysis 30
self-awareness 26–7
self-management 24–6, 38–40, 73,
    75, 137, 179
Senior, B. 13, 67
service 136
sexist abuse 33
sexual abuse 51, 52, 62
sexual relationships 59, 160
sexual stereotypes 45
sexuality 26, 58–64, 191
shared responsibility xiv, 78–80, 103
Sheffield 181
sideboard 95
sleep in 112
smell 5–6, 147
smoking 117–21
social services committee 20
socio-technical system(s) 124–7
Southwark College xv
staff groups 108–9, 145; Black, gay
    and lesbian, women's 34, 108
staff selection 72, 133
Staffing in Residential Homes 112
staffing levels 112, 150
starting work 23
Stirling, J. 90
stories 52, 164, 165
subculture 12, 118, 192
superintendent 18, 85
Supermanager 80–4
supermarket 176
supervision 9, 26, 31, 36, 59, 70, 86,
    87, 105–8, 109–11, 145, 151–2,
    154
supper 53, 55
system(s) 145; *see also*
    socio-technical systems

task 100; primary 4, 125–43, 146, 190
Task Force (Pensioner's Link) xiv
Tavistock Clinic xv
teacher 68
teddy bear 53
teenagers, late nights 54
television 55, 115
tenants 21
theory 42
therapeutic communication 49, 56, 57

therapeutic community 163
therapeutic relationship(s) 8
therapeutic work 53
time management 39
time off 111, 113
'to do' list 39
training and development 109–11, 186
transference 42, 46
transport 177–8
Trist, E. and Bamforth, K. 124
tucking in 53
Tulse Hill School xiv

unconscious forces 83, 169; motivation 30, 69; responses 49
unions 133, 134, 141, 151, 180

Utting, W. 64
unprofessional conduct 61

violence 10, 12–3, 52, 64–7, 129, 165, 166
vision 72–3, 169
visitor(s) 99, 147
volunteer(s) 98

Wagner Report 169, 182
Warwickshire 172
Watt, S. 87
Westland, P. 87
White society 7, 165
Wilson, M. 91
Winnicott, D. 86, 148
workload, limits 17